PRENATAL EXPOSURE
TO DRUGS/ALCOHOL

ABOUT THE AUTHOR

Jeanette M. Soby's educational background includes a BA in Psychology and a MS in Education from Portland State University in Portland, Oregon.

Her professional career in education began in 1970, working with children diagnosed as schizophrenic and autistic. Later positions included teaching and academic evaluation of youngsters, from all grades, with the full spectrum of learning disabilities found in public school students. She conducts workshops for school districts, and courses on prenatal exposure to drugs and alcohol, through various universities, for educators and specialists working with this population.

Jeanette M. Soby has served as a Citizen Review Board (CRB) Chair for the Oregon Supreme Court, reviewing cases of children who have been removed from their biological families. This service on the CRB has provided her with experience in the social and community problems related to substance abuse.

Second Edition

PRENATAL EXPOSURE TO DRUGS/ALCOHOL

Characteristics and Educational Implications of Fetal Alcohol Syndrome and Cocaine/Polydrug Effects

By

JEANETTE M. SOBY

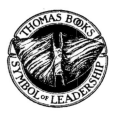

CHARLES C THOMAS • PUBLISHER, LTD.
Springfield • Illinois • U.S.A.

Published and Distributed Throughout the World by

CHARLES C THOMAS • PUBLISHER, LTD.
2600 South First Street
Springfield, Illinois 62704

© 2006 by CHARLES C THOMAS • PUBLISHER, LTD.

ISBN 0-398-07634-0 (hard)
ISBN 0-398-07635-9 (paper)

Library of Congress Catalog Card Number: 2005055943

With THOMAS BOOKS *careful attention is given to all details of manufacturing
and design. It is the Publisher's desire to present books that are satisfactory as to their
physical qualities and artistic possibilities and appropriate for their particular use.*
THOMAS BOOKS *will be true to those laws of quality that assure a good name
and good will.*

Printed in the United States of America
SM-R-3

Library of Congress Cataloging-in-Publication Data

Soby, Jeanette M.
   Prenatal exposure to drugs/alcohol : characteristics and educational impli-
cations of fetal alcohol syndrome and cocaine/polydrug effects / by Jeanette
M. Soby.--2nd ed.
     p. cm.
   Includes bibliographical references and index.
   ISBN 0-398-07634-0 -- ISBN 0-398-07635-9 (pbk.)
   1. Children of prenatal substance abuse--Education--United States. 2.
Children of prenatal substance abuse--United States. 3. Child development-
-United States. I. Title.

LC4806.4.S63 2006
371.91'6--dc22

                                  2005055943

PREFACE

This book describes the characteristics of youngsters effected by prenatal drug/alcohol exposure and explores strategies to circumvent this damage, maximizing the individual's remaining strengths. Information and suggestions are primarily for the professionals in education who can provide supportive coordination for caregivers, mental health, and medical service providers; in terms of relaying information and pinpointing techniques for learning that are the most successful for each youngster.

Medical literature on the physical, cognitive, and behavioral characteristics of this population is described for readers without a medical background. Terminology commonly used by various disciplines, outside of education, is included generally as background to the continued investigations that this text hopefully inspires. Research related to aspects of learning, particularly relevant to deficiencies seen in this population, is included to provide the background necessary for the development of individual instructional strategies that cover the needs of both severely effected and moderately effected individuals. Discoveries about the organization and development of normal memory/ learning have been brought together from the disciplines of education, biology, sociology, speech, cognitive psychology, and the neurosciences. The combined strength of various disciplines help us take into consideration the child's total environment, prenatal and postnatal.

Scientific knowledge is advancing rapidly with technology adding to the velocity, new findings add to and integrate with older research or inspire new ways for us to understand. For example, early research found prenatal cocaine more damaging, based on studies that often did not rule out other drugs that can cause birth defects, teratogens, such as tobacco and alcohol.

A sampling of relevant studies are referenced as support and information detail. The combination of risk factors in the substance-abusing population have made it difficult for researchers to determine specific independent effects of prenatal exposure to a single drug, or a single event.

Advances in technology are opening windows previously unavailable, allowing researchers to see mental operations of the brain as it learns and remembers. Neuroimaging that locates which areas of the brain are damaged can more accurately influence our expectations for a youngster, while pointing to instructional strategies and adaptations. Neurophysiology, neurochemistry, and neuropsychology inform the field of behavioral teratology. Understanding the biology of learning provides us a foundation to inform current and future education. While neurologists are studying the location and functioning of the learning brain–educators are looking at what activities produce the fastest, most stable, long-term learning.

However, we must look at research as tentative knowledge that points to ways of looking at, of understanding; a beginning step toward remediation design. Yet, the definitive statements we want from research are, only directions–qualified directions.

Children damaged from prenatal exposure to drugs/alcohol have been in the classroom all along, with teachers providing them an education. This text looks to educators who have found successful instructional techniques for use with students exhibiting many of the same physical, intellectual, and behavioral characteristics as students with effects from prenatal exposure to alcohol or cocaine/polydrugs. Educational needs, successful learning environments, and instructional techniques are addressed. Yet, despite medical, educational, and social support, most children with brain damage caused by prenatal alcohol exposure retain their handicaps throughout life. Thus, the environment must be adapted to optimize the experiences of these youngsters, because brain damage has removed much of their flexibility to use cognitive strategies.

I've included theoretical positions regarding cognitive processes that relate to the practical demands of instruction and successful skill acquisition. Unavoidably, the theoretical interpretations and topics presented dealing with learning are biased by my experience. I have made an effort to keep some reasonably concise parameters on the aspects of learning and instructional strategies that fit the range of needs presented by youngsters damaged from prenatal drug exposure.

Research and experience have provided such an extensive base of information I'm sure my indebtedness to some sources will go unacknowledged. Articles I have read and conversations that became so much a part of me, I no longer recognize an idea is not my own. I weave together medical research on maternal drug use and subsequent child health, with cognitive research focused on learning to inform remedial instructional possibilities. Areas of concern are touched on: attachment, infant-stimulation, communication, the cognitive processes involved in learning, instructional techniques, learning environments. Questions brought up during my lectures are included in this edition.

Some information is included as a reference point to where inquiry is headed. Whereas, many studies have been done on prenatal exposure to alcohol, after doctors David Smith and Kenneth Jones published in 1973, studies of other prenatal drug exposures, such as marijuana, are not as abundant. Why? Maybe funding has not been available, maybe there is limited interest in the answer, or damage is not considered significant enough to study.

Youngsters born with drug effects resulting from maternal use of alcohol have a medical diagnostic label. At a summit hosted by the National Organization of Fetal Alcohol Syndrome (NOFAS), April 2004, a consensus statement regarding diagnostic terminology was made "Fetal Alcohol Spectrum Disorders (FASD) is an umbrella term describing the range of effects that can occur in an individual whose mother drank alcohol during pregnancy. These effects may include physical, mental, behavioral, and/or learning disabilities with possible lifelong implications for problems in many areas of life: work, school, and social relations. The term FASD is not intended for use as a clinical diagnosis" (www.nofas.org). The umbrella term FASD will be used to represent Fetal Alcohol Syndrome (FAS), Partial FAS, Fetal Alcohol Effects (FAE), prenatal alcohol effects (PAE), alcohol-related birth defects (ARBD), alcohol-related neurodevelopmental disorder (ARND), and alcohol exposed static encephalopathy, throughout this book.

Diagnostic labels describing specific characteristics of impairments have not been attached to other drugs such as cocaine, heroine, marijuana, or other newer "designer drugs." The primary focus of the medical research included here is on alcohol and cocaine. Addictive maternal behavior for drugs other than alcohol often involves polysubstance abuse, use of a variety of drugs. Although not a medical diagnosis, the term *Fetal Drug Effects* (FDE) will be used to describe youngsters manifesting possible drug effects from prenatal cocaine and polydrug exposure, with cocaine the primary drug used, except when references to effects from a specific drug need to be delineated.

Looking at prenatal fetal cocaine/polydrug exposure, the consistent theme emerging is a correlation with subtle decrements in measures of cognitive development; sustained attention, arousal, and regulation of responses to stress. The popular media predictions of catastrophic life outcomes and effects on offspring in the late 1980s failed to evaluate the physiologic research results in light of maternal-fetal health problems and psychosocial risks that can accompany severe addictions to alcohol, cocaine, tobacco, and other drugs. The cumulative risk of disadvantaged social and environmental circumstances, compound biological frailties. This confluence of events contribute to an infant's poorer functioning; inadequate parenting, social isolation, maltreatment, domestic violence, and poverty.

The book falls into three sections. Part one presents the characteristics of youngsters prenatally drug exposed, giving the reader an understanding of possible damage. Part two presents background on the cognitive processes involved in learning. The primary focus of this section is on normal learning processes. Understanding normal cognitive processes allows the reader to extrapolate based on how a specific youngster is functioning. Part three describes instructional strategies, for the learning and everyday life experiences youngsters with disabilities find challenging.

In addition to medical and education research, information came from my work with families, community services, the judicial system, and education services. Experiences were derived from my work in the field of special education, from my service on the Citizen Review Board for the Oregon Justice Department, and from interviews with medical foster moms, teachers, social workers, nurses, other service and care providers, together with parents. I have also used experiences from professionals in the field who attended my course on prenatal exposure to drugs and alcohol. Working with the Juvenile Justice System and the Children Service Division, I reviewed placement and services for youngsters removed from their homes. Paternal substance abuse is frequently involved when children are removed from their homes due to neglect, physical abuse, and sexual abuse.

Interviews with Chris Amos, Joan Marguis, Robin Lindsley, Billie McKenzie, and Beth Caruso provide examples of successful instructional and management techniques. Interviewees included a social worker, a nurse, a school psychologist, and teachers employed in the Portland Public Schools, a small city community with an urban population enrollment of fifty-six thousand students.

Additional descriptions of hands-on experiences came from interviews with medical foster moms working with the Children's Services Division in Portland, Oregon. Some of the most down-to-earth heartfelt information came from interviews with medical foster moms, the moms that take medically high-risk drug effected newborns home from the hospital. Many of the moms' I talked to had histories devoted to child care, their own children, adopted children, and foster care children.

All the adults I interviewed report recognizing the need for them to consistently present a calm demeanor, and to make a conscious effort not to take the difficult behavior of these youngsters personally. Behavior that from a nonneurologically damaged youngster would mean malicious intent. Keeping a calm atmosphere was found to be a successful instruction/behavior management technique. All of the people interviewed had to continually work at accepting the youngsters' lack of social judgment.

Parents and educators need to recognize deficits primarily so that strategies can be found to circumvent these deficits. Instructional and management recommendations are made with this in mind.

J.M.S.

CONTENTS

PART I

ILLUSTRATIONS

PRENATAL EXPOSURE
TO DRUGS/ALCOHOL

PART I

Chapter 1

INTRODUCTION: WHAT IS THE PROBLEM?

Polydrug use, taking more than one drug, is typical for chemically addicted mothers. Commonly abused drugs during pregnancy include: alcohol, a depressant; marijuana, that overstimulates the sensory nerves of touch, taste, sight, and hearing; amphetamine, that stimulates; heroin that produces euphoria; morphine that produces euphoria; and cocaine that produces euphoria. A problem that is significant to both the offspring and society.

This chapter discusses risk and causal factors; the need for identification and multilevel intervention. Research cautions are presented, giving the reader a broader perspective to evaluate the research this book is based on, and the additional research sparked by interest.

INCIDENTS

The most widely used prevalence estimate of FAS, in the general United States population, is 1 to 1.5 cases per 100 live births. Also, mortality is about two thousand infant deaths in the U.S. from FAS and related disorders (Burd, Cotsonas-Hassler, Martsolf, and Kerbeshian 2003). In addition, the Centers of Disease Control (CDC) (2000), found about thirty percent of the women who knew they were pregnant, reported alcohol consumption. Youngsters who have not been diagnosed have not been counted. Maternal substance abuse crosses all social levels, however, doctors frequently do not look for subtle signs of alcohol or cocaine exposure in babies born full term that appear healthy. Thus, rates may be low. Incidences of FASD for

different ethnic groups derived from the Birth Defects Monitoring
Program of the CDC show Native Americans are at the highest risk
with 29.9 per 10,000 births, varying with different tribes (Chavez,
Cordero, and Becerra 1989). These figures reflect American Indians
may be physiologically predisposed to alcoholism because of deficits
in the ability to metabolize acetaldehyde, a product of alcohol degra-
dation. This may add to the misperception that American Indians
drink more alcohol (only 42% of adult Navajo Indians drink alcohol)
than other ethnic groups (Carney and Chermak 1991).

Medically needy babies require longer hospital stays with increased overall hospital costs. The additional medical costs for
drug/alcohol exposed newborns, at the national level have been estimated in the billions. These cost estimates do not include the lifespan
support resources needed. For example, the medical foster parents and
extended families who care for these children need respite care and
parent training. The financial and profound social costs of this problem demand public health involvement in prevention, drug treatment,
prenatal care, and educational services.

A recurrent theme stated by medical, judicial, and educational professionals providing services to youngsters is that "kids are different
now than they were ten years ago." Drug use changes people, changes
society. Today's problems are different; thus, solutions must be different. No matter how dedicated teachers are, how good schools are, a
great education *is not as good as a bad family*. The families' impact is
paramount. During a discussion of these concerns with medical and
education providers, a prekindergarten teacher's sincere remark cap-
tured the fears, compassion, and hopelessness this social problem
evokes, "At the end of the school day when I have two or three children who do not want to leave, it's scary to me." What kind of home
are these youngsters avoiding? The life experiences some of these
youngsters are exposed to suggest that a safe home is an anomaly
rather than the norm. Teachers work hard to provide safety, structure,
and control during school hours; then many students go home to
chaotic environments. Children prenatally exposed to drugs/alcohol
may have had lots of adults coming in and out of their lives: parents,
relatives, foster care, and a variety of service providers. They may not
ever have had a stable adult in their life.

> At the end of the school day when I have two or three children who do not want to leave; it's scary to me (pre-kindergarten teacher).

ADDICTION LIFESTYLE–RISK FACTORS

These children can be impacted by a group of risk factors: chaotic lifestyle, violence, abuse, neglect, being raised by brothers and sisters who are children themselves, and multiple placements with relatives or foster care. The parent-child relationships of youngsters living with parents expose them to the maternal personality disorders that flourish with drug use. Disruption and chaos describe the households of chemically addicted parents who have a commitment to chemicals, not to their children. As addiction worsens, the procurement of drugs becomes consuming; substances of abuse take precedent over all other considerations, including maternal and fetal health, nothing but the drug has any significance (Gawin 1991; MacGregor, Do, Keith, Bachicha, and Chasnoff 1989). ". . . Addictive drugs not only modify behavior but the brain itself . . ." (Restak 1988). Brain reward systems involved in the reinforcing effects of drugs of abuse promote drug use behavior, cocaine addicts report that all thoughts center on cocaine during binges. Disregard of the child's needs, neglect and abuse, follow parental addiction. These addicted, hopeless, scared mothers under the influence of mind-altering drugs, need care themselves.

Adult lifestyle is intimately tied to child development and familial relationships. How will the alcohol or cocaine addicted mother be able to take care of an addicted baby that is likely to have ongoing medical and educational needs? Can the alcoholic mother provide a safe and nurturing home for the child with FASD? When getting high is of prime importance, can a drug addicted mother, living in a chaotic drug environment care for and cope with the frustrations of an inconsolable infant with shakes and a sharp piercing cry? Will this mother be alert to the medical needs of a fragile infant? Inconsistent and intermittent nurturing may come from parents or caregivers who are emotionally needy themselves.

Youngsters may be exposed to unpredictable environments with parents coming in and out of their lives; at risk for multiple placements and multiple caregivers. Many of the mothers with chronic addictions do not live long enough to raise their children. Foster care placement, often multiple, provides the family environment for many of these fragile youngsters who require multiple educational and health care services. Prenatal drug/alcohol exposure can cause a wide range of impairments which are mitigated or exacerbated by the child's early environment. Not one of the eight children in the Los Angeles School District pilot project kindergarten class, for youngsters damaged by prenatal drug exposure, lives with his or her biological mother. Some children have been in as many as eight different homes. Most of the children are being reared by foster parents or grandparents (Trost 1989).

Maternal drug use may spread for generations resulting in a multi-generational cycle of drug addition. The risks of drug use compound rather than remain limited to just the specific days used taking drugs. A medical foster care mom wonders "were their parents alcoholic and their grandparents also? How many generations?"

PREVENTION

Prospective mothers might not recognize that their life style, especially drug/alcohol use and abuse, can have unintended harmful consequences on the outcome of their newborn. Consequences that can impact the child's whole life, putting intellectual and social opportunities at peril. Women in their childbearing years and pregnant women might choose not to use alcohol or other drugs if they were informed about the detrimental consequences that drug/alcohol use can have on a fetus: consequences that can persist into adulthood.

The mother most likely to jeopardize her pregnancy with drug use and give birth to an infant with FASD/FDE may be a victim of FASD herself. Because of her limited abstract thinking, she cannot understand the serious effects drug/alcohol use during pregnancy can have on her child. Without multilevel intervention involving a partnership of services, prenatally drug/alcohol effected newborns could be in the next generation of parents with effected offspring (Dorris 1989; Clarren 2005). In addition to the poor judgment risk of mothers with FASD, a genetic bias toward alcoholism may exist.

Educators found drug use prevention activities, including teaching parents-to-be about the influence of drug/alcohol abuse on the developing fetus, most effective with students nongenetically susceptible to addiction. Teachers in both middle and high school, report using a strategy based on "others" problems rather than the student's own, to be the most successful of all the prevention curriculum activities. Students' write a paper or make a list of problems people they know, who are using drugs/alcohol, are having. Based on this activity, genuine "real-life" class discussions have taken place. Remnants of old antidrug strategies, exaggerating the effects of drugs, which led to a loss of credibility, remain today.

Doctor Lemoine's early observations of children of alcoholic mothers in 1967, found that 5 alcoholic mothers, who after giving up drinking gave birth to one or more normal babies (Lemoine 2003; Koren, Nulman, Chudley, and Loocke 2003). During a workshop at a private school, the teachers discussed a mother who had given birth to eight children with FASD, she stopped drinking and gave birth to a child who did not have FASD. In agreement with this, Korkman, Kettunen, and Autti-Ramo (2003) found "If pregnant mothers are able to stop drinking even as late as in trimester II, the risk of negative cognitive sequelae is considerably reduced."

IDENTIFICATION

Parents may not be aware their newborn has unique needs. Early identification alerts parents and service providers, so appropriate care for an infant's development and health care needs can be given. A contrasting opinion regarding drug exposure, was expressed in the January, 1992 issue of *Journal of the American Medical Association*, commentary section. Doctors were concerned that labeling youngsters prenatally exposed to cocaine, as having irremediable damage, would result in fewer services provided for these children because expectations would be so low (Mayes, Granger, Bornstein, and Zuckerman 1992). Although labeling has the potential for negative consequences, accurate expectations based on early identification are likely to have a positive affect on the child's life (Streissguth et al. 2004). Identification of FASD is complicated, youngsters are usually seen by a pediatrician, then referred to a dysmorphologist for a thorough diagnosis. Stoler and Holmes (2000) recommend obstetricians provide medical records to pediatricians, to help alert early identification. The ability to intervene early in the child's life is based on diagnosis. Doctors' Streissguth and Kanter (1999) use the term "secondary disabilities" to describe FASD problems, that are a consequence of "primary" deficits in cognition, communication, and learning; which can impact social competence. This complex nature-nurture relationship between biology and environmental factors on development, is the reasoning for early intervention.

Early diagnosis ensures youngsters will not miss the benefits of early intervention and access to multidisciplinary child development teams. Poitra and colleagues (2003) found a community/school-based screening program had a 95 percent accuracy rate, and screening took less than 15 minutes per child. Ashley, Stachowiak, Clarren, and Clausen (2002) looked at the incidence of FASD in the foster care population using the *FAS DPN Facial Photographic Screening Tool* which was developed for assessment of photographs on a computer monitor. Screenings took approximately 10 minutes per child. They found the prevalence of FASD was 10 to 15 times greater than in the general population (Astley et al. 2002). Other maternal report screening tools, one using three to four questions about maternal alcohol use was able to identify offspring at highest risk for FASD; hence, directing the youngsters to a complete medical evaluation (Barr and Streissguth 2001).

An infant care specialist, a school nurse, and others interviewed, who are concerned with identifying youngsters with FASD/FDE, find parents to be very poor historians. Identification of youngsters, by means of self-reported maternal histories suffer from parental reluctance to admit to either drug/alcohol use or the amount and frequency of use. A nurse for a head start program has found a way around parents who understate their youngsters prenatal drug exposure. With nonjudgmental assertiveness, when taking the child's history, she asks if the child demonstrated any of the symptoms of withdrawal, specifically asking if as a newborn the child, was startled easily, had a high-pitched cry, poor suck, seizures, tight muscles, interest in the human face, and so on. She has found that parents are more likely to answer these questions honestly. She walks the parents' through examples of a variety of day-to-day routines and early milestones. As the child's past history is reviewed, patterns may be discovered that help explain current behaviors, areas of strength, needs, and perceptual uniqueness.

Table 1. Basic Functioning History.

Medical problems/history
Bedtime, sleeping awakening
Temperament
Independent coping behaviors
Self-care skills
Chores/responsibilities
Skills/talents
Play skills/behaviors
Adult relationships
Peer relationships
Unusual behaviors

ALCOHOL METABOLISM: FETAL RISK

Alcohol metabolism takes place in the liver, where alcohol is initially oxidized to acetaldehyde, by alcohol dehydrogenase (ADH), this toxic acetaldehyde is then metabolized, by mitochondrial aldehyde dehydrogenase (ALDH2), to acetate. Genes involved in alcohol metabolism: genes that effect functional ADH and ALDH activities may influence the risk of alcoholism. Genes that effect alcohol drinking behavior: the quantity and frequency of alcohol consumption.

Maternal consumption of the teratogen alcohol during pregnancy is the cause of FASD, the most common nongenetic cause of mental retardation. Yet, not all women who use alcohol during pregnancy have offspring with FASD. Genetic differences may be predictors. Researchers are looking at alleles (variations of a gene) of the alcohol metabolizing enzyme gene ADH2, as predictors of FASD. Studies of different alleles of the ADH2 gene show differing results (Chambers and Jones 2002). The ADH2*3 allele, found primarily in Africans, is associated with rapid metabolism of alcohol, possibly enzymes more efficiently metabolize alcohol at high blood alcohol concentrations (Eriksson et al. 2001). The ADH2*2 allele was found to be more common in mothers who did not have offspring with FASD, suggesting the ADH2*2 may contribute protection against FASD (Viljoen et al. 2001).

The implication is that there is a genetic potential of a person to metabolize alcohol which may reduce or promote excessive alcohol use; thus, increasing the risk of FASD for offspring or of having a protective effect (Jones 2003). Continued research may help us predict, which maternal genotype, which women who drink alcohol, are at the highest risk of having an effected child.

Francis Collins and Craig Venter, two principle genome sequencers for the Human Genome Project; published in 2001, a sequence of the human genome. Personality trait variations related to alcoholism, are found to be from combinations of many genes rather than one single gene. For example, a high interest in novelty-seeking impulsive behaviors, along with a low interest in harm avoidance uninhibited behaviors (Cloninger, Sigvardsson, and Bohman 1996). Scientists are in the early stages of understanding the genetic contribution to susceptibility for alcoholism, looking at how and when different genes work together.

PATERNAL CONTRIBUTION

FASD is caused by maternal drinking, not fathers. Researchers have found conflicting results concerning lower birth weight on the offspring of fathers who consumed alcohol before conception. In general, the newborns' risk of behavior and cognitive deficits increase as the birth weight decreases. Low birth weight is commonly accepted as $5^1/2$ pounds; very low birth weight as $2^1/4$ pounds. Little and Sing (1986) found that infants of fathers who drank two drinks a day had offspring that weighed about a half a pound less than offspring of fathers who did not. Conflicting findings were produced by other researchers who did not find that paternal drinking before conception and during their partners pregnancy resulted in lower birth weight for offspring (Savitz, Zhang, Schwingl, and John 1992; Passaro, Little, Savitz, and Noss 1998). Damaged sperm may cause spontaneous abortion, Mother Nature's first defense, often before the mother is aware of her pregnancy. Future research may find a paternal genetic contribution; possibly influencing if or how much the fetus is protected or vulnerable to maternal alcohol consumption.

RESEARCH EVALUATION CAUTION

Particular disciplines investigate different aspects of a subject: a social scientist sees the world through different eyes than a neurologist. Cautions are many, the title and the discussion section of a published study may suggest a more encompassing attribute than the results support or that the methods used measure. The researcher may have a personal or discipline-related emotional investment that can lead to an overemphasis of the importance of their findings. Hence, Montori and colleagues (2004) recommend reading the methods and results sections only. They also caution graphs can be misleading, for example, comparing different time frames to harms and benefits. Studies flawed by uncontrolled or unexamined potential variables: differences in sample characteristics and size, faulty comparisons, small treatment effects, examination of moderating characteristics, relevancy of sub-group analyses, as well as the degree of statistical control, can lead to differing conclusions. Different agendas = different conclusions. These methodologic limitations fuel the fire of research disagreements.

Subjects recruited from a population referred to clinics are often used in the studies cited in this book. Clinic subjects are likely to be in a low socioeconomic risk factor group and also may be associated with high developmental risk without drug/alcohol exposure. Studies may exclude offspring of mothers who are very seriously addicted and mothers who's doctors haven't questioned them regarding drug use. People with congenital malformations or other more disabling conditions, or individuals with milder symptoms who can cover or compensate, may not be represented in the studies used. Control groups may come from families with multiple life stressors, such as brief homelessness and changes in the primary caregiver. Subjects for each study possesses a unique constellation of variables, and the degree of statistical control varies widely from study to study.

Many investigators have turned to animal models; both to reduce the conflicting findings of and to inform human studies, and to determine exactly what are the causal factors. Is there a connection between prenatal drug exposure and the birth defects seen in humans? Animal studies provide models of outcome based on control of exposure and timing. Patterns of dosage levels can be isolated to the prenatal period and isolated to a specific drug exposure. Drug administration protocols offer control of dosage level, other drugs used, and nutrition. No measure of drug/alcohol exposure is completely accurate, extrapolation from animal study data to effects on children has limitations, yet provides direction.

Mayes (2003) offers key principles to evaluate research questions on the relationship between a prenatal toxin exposure and later developmental impairment (1) what are the possible mechanisms of effect, (2) what is the specific teratogenic agent or event, (3) the timing of exposure, (4) what are the possible dose-response relations, (5) what are the most likely outcomes related to the mechanisms of action of the exposure, (6) when are outcomes most likely to be apparent, and (7) what conditions ameliorate or exacerbate exposure-related functional outcomes. How does the teratogenic exposure, disruption of process x affect other maturational processes?

Studies may not be designed in ways that fully reveal children's capabilities. Tasks used to measure a skill may not isolate that skill. For example, results of a test using pictures rather than words may provide a result too narrow in scope, a result that statistical controls do not adjust for. Although I advise the reader of research to be skeptical, I, too, may have accepted as factual only possibilities.

Chapter 2

PRENATAL DRUG/ALCOHOL EXPOSURE

The primary drugs of abuse with the possibility of a teratogenic effect producing anomalies in offspring are alcohol and cocaine. A description of the intellectual, physical, and behavioral characteristics of youngsters with a diagnosis of FASD and youngsters prenatally exposed to other drugs, based on medical research, is presented in this chapter. There is no typical profile, the continuum of impairments range from mild to severe.

THE FETAL ENVIRONMENT

Any drug that crosses the blood-brain barrier and has an effect on the central nervous system of the mother also crosses the placenta, affecting both maternal and fetal circulation. The placenta separates the circulatory systems of the fetus and the mother, transferring substances from the mother to the fetus. For example, as a result of the placenta's metabolic activity, which is separate from the mother's, cocaine is changed into a less active metabolite; hence, providing a moderate degree of protection for the fetus (Beaconsfield, Birdwood, and Beaconsfield 1980; Roe, Little, Bawdon, and Gilstrap 1990).

Many drugs involved in maternal substance abuse are *teratogens*, drugs that in certain dosages can cause birth defects. The word teratogen is derived from the Greek word "Terato" which means literally, "to make monsters." Teratogens have a long lag period; it may take ten years after birth for all the effects of the drug to show up. For example, the academic demands and social expectations for an adolescent

15

may expose deficits not previously identified.

Variable fetal effects can be partially accounted for by individual differences in drug metabolism, and that drugs are slowly metabolized by the immature fetus. The original drug and the metabolites of that drug remain in the amniotic fluid much longer than in the mother. "Moreover, generally speaking the fetus is exposed to the same drugs, food additives and environmental pollutants that the pregnant mother is exposed to" (Beaconsfield et al. 1980). Cocaine metabolites were found in newborns' urine 96 hours after birth, when maternal use was one to two days before delivery (Van de Bor, Walther, and Ebrahimi 1990). Cocaine may be present in the mother from 24 to 48 hours after use, while metabolites remain in the neonate from four to six days (Burkett, Yasin, and Palow 1990; Johanson and Fischman 1989; Peters and Theorell 1991). Both mother and fetus may have increased and prolonged exposure and toxicity to cocaine due to altered metabolism during pregnancy (Gingras, Weese-Mayer, Hume, and O'Donnell 1992).

The main intoxicant in alcoholic beverages is ethyl alcohol, a relatively simple organic chemical made up of carbon, oxygen, and hydrogen, that is soluble in both water and fat. The fetus lacks an enzyme, known as *alcohol dehydrogenase*, which is responsible for metabolizing alcohol. Because the fetal liver and kidneys are immature, drugs are slow to be broken down and excreted. Thus, the level of alcohol can build up in the fetus, particularly in the brain.

Is there a safe amount of alcohol for a pregnant woman to consume? No. But not all women who drink alcohol during their pregnancy have offspring with FASD, the individual health of the mother and the gestational stage of alcohol consumption play an important part. Although researchers do not agree on a safe amount, 1.5 drinks per day have been found to be associated with a high incidence of FAS (Autti-Ramo 2002). Olson and colleagues (1997) found subtle alcohol related neuropsychological deficits in offspring, exposed to even maternal 'social drinking' levels, that were consistent with behavioral dysfunction seen in youngsters prenatally exposed to higher doses of alcohol: deficits in sustained attention, response inhibition, spatial memory, and variability in task performance. Willford, Richardson, Leech, and Day (2004) also found memory processing deficits in both recall and recognition memory for verbal memory of word-pairs, in offspring of mothers who engaged in moderate drinking. In addition, it was found that a pattern of maternal continuous use, even in doses considerably below one drink per day, resulted in growth deficits for their offspring (Day et al. 2002). Even at low levels of prenatal exposure, mild deficits can disrupt vital social and intellectual life potential for offspring.

RISK FACTORS

Multiple factors can adversely impact the fetus of a pregnant chemically addicted woman: inadequate nutrition, drug/nutrition interactions, lack of prenatal care, maternal age, maternal physical and mental health, exposure to infections in utero, fetal genetic susceptibility, in addition to interactions with other drugs, drug use amounts and frequency of use, together with the contaminants used to adulterate street drugs. Also, the prenatal effects of drug exposure may be exacerbated by social factors, such as, family dysfunction, environmental deprivation, lack of prenatal care. If a genetically transmitted behavior disorder of minimal brain dysfunction or FASD contributed to a mother

Table 2. Factors Impacting the Fetus of a Pregnant Substance-Abusing Woman.

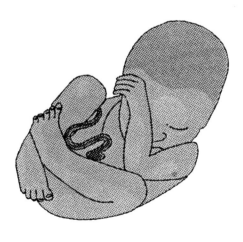

• Poor maternal nutrition

• Lack of prenatal care

• Maternal age

• Maternal health

• Fetal genetic susceptibility

• Gestational stage of drug exposure

• Drug factors
  Dose
    Type and frequency of use
    The way drugs are used
      a) mixed of one drug at a time
      b) injected
      c) smoked (free-base)
      d) sniffing
    Contaminants used to adulterate street
      drugs
    Characteristics of the drugs and their
      metabolites

becoming a drug/alcohol abuser in the first place, the risks to her off-spring may be even more complex than maternal drug use alone. Maternal disabilities are likely to negatively aggravate nonbiological aspects of prenatal and postnatal care.

Potential fetal damage associated with cocaine exposure from vaso-constriction may occur at any point in gestation as well as in early pregnancy (Hoyme et al. 1990). Offspring of mothers, over 30 years of age, using drugs/alcohol were twice as likely to fall below the 10th percentile in height and weight (Covington, Nordstrom-Klee, Ager, Sokol, and Delaney-Black 2002). Maternal age, over 30 years, has been shown to influence fetal susceptibility to the long term effects of intrauterine growth retardation: small-for-gestational-age (SGA) infants, are at risk for long term growth impairments, cognitive deficits, and perinatal and neonatal mortality (O'Shea et al. 1997).

Maternal Health

The fetus can be exposed to the teratogenic effects of drugs/alco-hol during the critical period of organogenesis, before the mother real-izes she is pregnant. The effects that specific drugs have depend upon maternal health, the genetic makeup of the fetus, the developmental stage of the fetus at the time of exposure, along with the characteristics of the drug used. For example, the interaction of cocaine on nutrition, can produce a temporary period of anorexia. Along with drug terato-gens, drug/nutrition interactions that contribute to maternal under-nourishment may have a significant detrimental effect on offspring. Nelson, Lerner, Needlman, Salvator, and Singer (2004) found children prenatally cocaine-exposed, who had iron-deficiency anemia, had a two-fold decrease in full scale Intelligent Quotient (IQ) scores.

There is a high prevalence of psychiatric illness among adult sub-stance abusers, for women rates are particularly elevated for antisocial disorders, post-traumatic stress, mania, schizophrenia, and major de-pression (Kessler et al. 1996). Singer, Salvator, and colleagues (2002) found maternal psychological distress in addition to cocaine/polydrug exposure related to poorer growth on head circumference for off-spring, which is an indicator of brain growth and cognitive develop-ment.

Maternal drugs/alcohol use often occur along with other risks to offspring: parental physical and mental health problems, social-voca-tional-education problems, and multigenerational family dysfunction.

Gestational Stages

The stage of embryonic or fetal development during which expo-sure to a drug occurs, determines which anatomic system is effected. The effects seen in the child depend on the amount and duration of drug/alcohol exposure.

Existing or developing structures can be disrupted, malformations of the brain and vital organs can result from insult during the embry-onic phase, from about the second through the eighth week. For exam-ple, drug exposure during the third week of embryonic development has the most harmful effect on the central nervous system and the heart. Development of crainofacial features and the forebrain occur from approximately weeks four through ten. Drug exposure during the seventh week has the most severe effect on the development of the arms, eyes, legs, teeth, palate, external genitalia, and the ears. Drug exposure during the second through the twelfth week has the most severe effect on facial formations (Astley, Clarren, Little, Sampson, and Daling 1992; Moore and Persaud 1993). Few developing systems escape harm when the mother drinks alcohol throughout the preg-nancy.

FETAL ALCOHOL SPECTRUM DISORDERS: FASD

"Behold, thou shalt conceive and bear a son; and now drink no wine or strong drink" (Judges 13:7). Medical research indicating that maternal alcohol consumption might affect offspring was published in the United States by Doctors' David Smith and Kenneth Jones in 1973, as a cluster of congenital birth defects linked with maternal alcohol consumption. Alcohol and its metabolites have the potential to cause physiologic and neurologic disturbances in fetal development. The probability of having a child with FASD increases with the amount and frequency of alcohol consumed. The severity of FASD is corre-lated with the amount of alcohol the mother consumes. Consumption

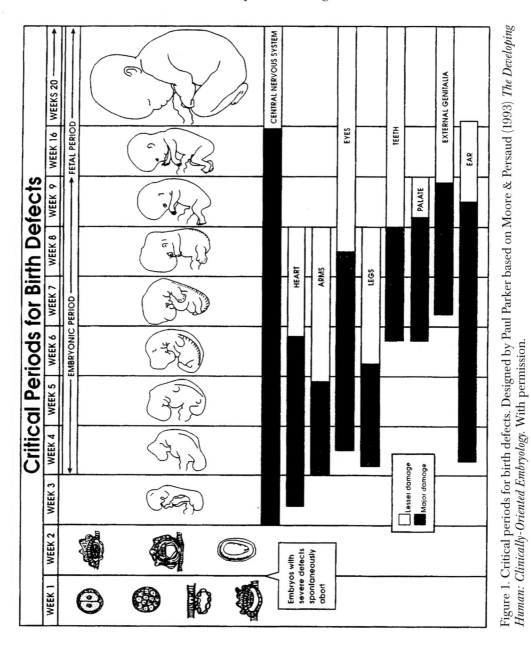

Figure 1. Critical periods for birth defects. Designed by Paul Parker based on Moore & Persaud (1993) *The Developing Human: Clinically-Oriented Embryology*. With permission.

of two or more ounces of alcohol per day, early in the pregnancy, was found to be associated with FASD like facial features (Astley et al. 1992). The severity of the physical characteristics of FASD determine the possibility of successful remediation and skill acquisition. As early as 1967, in France, Doctor Paul Lemoine published a discussion of 127 cases of children of alcoholic parents (Lemoine 2003).

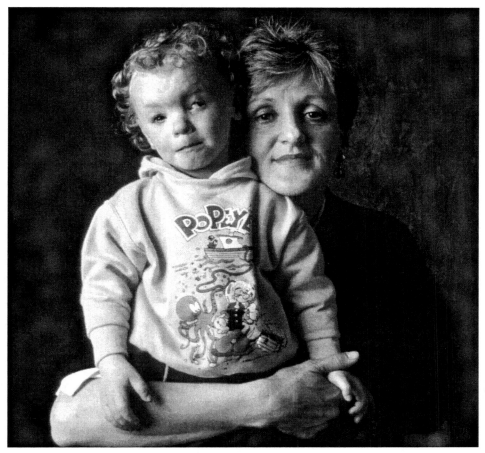

Figure 2. Fetal Alcohol Syndrome: Mother and child. (Photograph by George Steinmetz.)

Ernhart and colleagues (1987) looked at data from 359 neonates of mothers with alcohol use problems, and found a clear dose response relationship between embryonic and fetal alcohol exposure and anatomic congenital abnormalities. The range of characteristics that make up FAS include facial anomalies, growth deficiency, and mental retardation (Jones and Smith 1973; Streissguth, Sampson, and Barr 1989). Fetal Alcohol Effects (FAE) is a less severe version of FAS, milder or fewer FAS characteristics are seen in FAE (Jones, Smith, Ulleland, and Streissguth 1973).

Astley and Clarren (1999) developed a *Diagnostic Guide for Fetal Alcohol Syndrome and Related Conditions*, primarily to assist health care professionals. A diagnosis is based on key *sentinel* finding for growth and facial characteristics, and unchanging brain abnormalities, *static encephalopathy*: these characteristics are grouped into 22 diagnostic categories that help narrow the scope and pinpoint possible damage. Growth deficits, facial dysmorphology, and brain damage are characteristics required for a diagnosis of FAS: in addition to knowledge of maternal alcohol consumption.

Table 3. FASD Diagnostic Criteria.

FETAL ALCOHOL SPECTRUM DISORDER
- Characteristic pattern of facial anomalies
- Growth retardation
- Central Nervous System neurodevelopmental abnormalities
- Known history of maternal alcohol consumption

Characteristics: FASD

Children with FASD can have abnormalities in every part of their bodies. Prenatal or postnatal growth retardation can effect both body length and head circumference, resulting in premature birth and failure-to-thrive babies. They are born small and stay small. Deficits in weight, height, and head circumference, persist into adolescence (Day et al. 2002). Cranial/facial abnormalities include: small head circumference, flattened midface, small wide-set eyes, and drooping eyelids. Cardiovascular abnormalities include heart murmurs and malformations. Renal abnormalities include malformations and renal failure. In addition, there can be respiratory dysfunction, immune system dysfunction, and orthopedic abnormalities. Central nervous system dysfunction includes: *microencephaly* (small brain for body size), *hydrocephalus* (excess fluid in the cranium), and mental retardation. The broad range of neurological difficulties include speech and language disorders, learning disabilities, decreased attention span, tremulousness, weak grasp, head and body rocking, sleep disturbances, poor eye gaze, poor eye-hand coordination, *strabismus* (imbalanced eye muscles, one eye cannot focus with the other), and hearing impairments. "If any single one of the visual processing areas is damaged, the result is a specific impairment in perception" (Squire and Kandel 1999). Stromland and Hellstrom (1996) found 92 percent of the 25 children with FASD in Sweden who were referred to the Children's Hospital for significant eye problems also had significant ophthalmologic abnormalities. Many of the skeletal defects result from reduced intrauterine movement (Jones 2003). Swayze and colleagues (1997) found patients with the most severe facial dysmorphologic characteristics are more likely to have midline brain anomalies. In general, the greater the facial dysmorphology, the greater the degree of mental retardation.

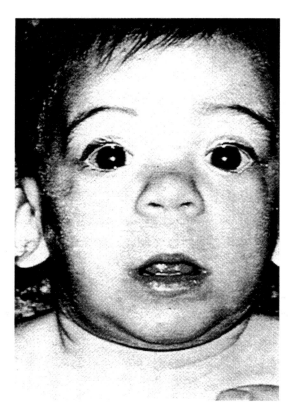

Unusual
Head Shape

Small Head
Circumference

Low Set Ears

Short Upturned
Nose
Sunken or Low
Nasal Bridge
Indistinct
Philtrum:
(Area Between
Nose and Upper
Lip Flattened or
Missing)

Eyes
Epicanthic Folds
(Eyelid Skin Folds
Protrude Over the
Inner Corner of
the Eye)
Short Palpebral
Fissures
(Short Eye Slits)

Face Looks Flat
Small Midface
Flat Cheeks

Thin Upper Lip

Figure 3. Fetal alcohol syndrome facial characteristics. The pattern of anomalies include the above facial features, growth deficiency, and mental retardation. Abnormalities are likely to occur in every part of the body. (Child diagnosed with FAS at nine months of age.)

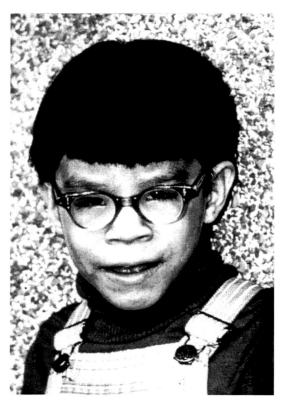

Figure 4. Child diagnosed with fetal alcohol syndrome at age five.

Developing Brain

"Further, it has become clear that the structure that is most sensitive to alcohol is the developing brain and that the resulting neurobehavioral abnormalities have the most profound and lasting consequences for affected individuals" (Jones 2003). The complexity of cortical circuitry, determines its functional capabilities. Brain imaging, magnetic resonance (MR) findings are contributing to understanding that brain dysmorphology is the center of the prenatal teratogenetic effect of alcohol. "It is the brain image, not the portrait, that is the more informative for these patients" (Bookstein, Streissguth, Sampson, Connor, and Barr 2002). The toxic effects of alcohol on the neurochemical and cellular elements of the developing brain are not simply global, some brain regions are more affected than others even within a given region. Alcohol alters neural development, the synthesis, release, receptor binding, and the signaling of a variety of neurotransmitters and neuromodulators. Neuropathology can include interference with cell division, proliferation, growth, differentiation, and migration of cells, along with the impairment of neurotransmitter systems.

Neuronal-glial interactions play a critical role throughout the ontogenetic process: cell generation, cell migration, and cellular maturation. Given that the corpus callosum is initially formed by bundles of glial cells, alterations of glial cells could be involved in the abnormalities of the corpus callosum. Findings of a research review by Guerri, Pascual, and Renau-Piqueras (2001), suggest in utero alcohol exposure induces structural and functional abnormalities in gliogenesis (geneses = origin) and glial-neuronal interactions. This review suggested that glial cells are a target of alcohol toxicity during brain development and may underlie neurodevelopmental abnormalities.

Sowell, Thompson, Mattson, and colleagues (2002) found brain shape abnormalities persist into adolescence. They speculate that cell maturational processes are effected: the continued depositing of myelin, from glial cells, during late brain development, up to 20 years after prenatal exposure to alcohol. In another study Sowell, Thompson, Peterson, and colleagues (2002) using voxel MRI's, three-dimensional brain images, found altered gray matter cortical surface asymmetry, in areas involved in language processing, and face recognition. Abnormalities in the outer layers of the left hemisphere were found that indicate dysmorphology beyond the overall microcephaly, smaller head size, seen in FASD (Sowell, Mattson, Thompson, et al. 2001).

Results from both structural and functional brain imaging show that although damage is diffuse, certain areas are more effected especially the limbic system: corpus callosum, hippocampus, basal ganglia, and the cerebellum. The caudate nucleus appears to account for most of the size reduction in the basal ganglia (Mattson, Schoenfeld, and Riley 2001). The basal ganglia is involved in the initiation and regulation of motor movement abilities and cognitive functions. The cerebellum is involved in control of posture, gait, balance, coordination, and learning. The hippocampus is involved in memory. The corpus callosum communicates information between the two hemispheres of the brain. Damage can alter the relationships between regions, resulting in problems with attention, intellectual and social functioning.

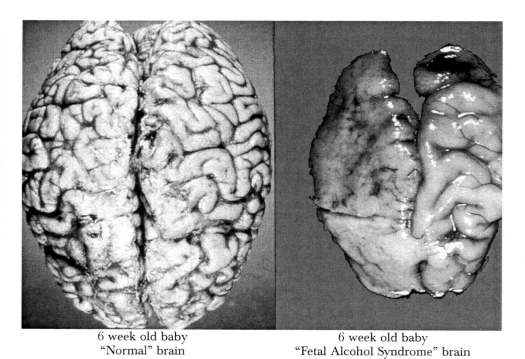

6 week old baby   6 week old baby
"Normal" brain   "Fetal Alcohol Syndrome" brain

Figure 5. Brain: Normal/FAS. Photo courtesy of Sterling Clarren MD.

Alcohol exposure can effect neuroanatomic size of the corpus callosum, ranging from small to complete agenesis (failure to develop), and location of the corpus callosum. Newer research-related verbal learning to corpus callosum location, more than size, or the facial anomalies, or the overall cognitive impairment of persons with FASD (Sowell, et al. 2001). MR scans revealed corpus callosum shape variations. A thick callosum was associated with deficits in executive function. A thin callosum was associated with deficits in motor function (Bookstein, Streissguth, et al. 2002). Given that callosal dysmorphology, for size and location, can exist in the absence of facial dysmorphology, diagnosis in the future, could be expanded.

Bookstein, Sampson, and colleagues (2002), looked at subjects age 14 to 37 and concluded, "The information from the corpus callosum and vicinity, as viewed in MR brain images of adolescent and adult subjects, may serve as a permanent record of the prenatal effects of alcohol, even in patients who are first suspected of these syndromes relatively late in life or who lack the facial signs of prenatal alcohol damage" (Bookstein et al. 2002).

Intellectual Functioning

"Mental retardation is a cardinal feature of FAS, and the syndrome, has emerged as the number one recognized disorder in which mental deficiency is a feature" (Abel 1984). Youngsters with FAS have IQ scores in the mildly retarded range, while those with FAE have, on average, IQ scores of 73 in the borderline range (Streissguth, LaDue, and Randels 1988). The mean IQ for youngsters with FAS is 68 with a range from 83 to below 58 (Streissguth, Randels, and Smith 1991). Individuals with FASD average a seven to nine-year-old functional intellectual level, with second to fourth grade academic skills (Streissguth, Aase, et al. 1991). FAS is the most common nongenetic cause of mental retardation. Intellectually, individuals with FASD range from severely retarded to well into the normal range. Their IQ scores remain, in general, fairly stable throughout life, with achievement scores lower than their IQ scores, also the biggest deficit is often in arithmetic functions (Streissguth and O'Malley 2000).

Cognitive deficits in attention, memory, and executive function reflect deficits beyond those measured by intelligence and achievement tests. Kerns, Don, Mateer, and Streissguth (1997) found, independent of IQ level: a higher performance IQ score than a verbal IQ score, with arithmetic lower than reading and spelling achievement. On psychological testing, the mean arithmetic standard scores have been found to be two-thirds of a standard deviation below mean IQ scores (Streissguth et al. 2004). Youngsters with FASD could do reading numbers and writing numbers, but had difficulty with number calculation and estimation tasks (Kopera-Frye, Dehaene, and Streissguth 1996). Number estimation tasks can reflect deficits in comprehension. For example, the estimation question "How many children can a schoolbus carry?" also involves comprehension.

Prenatally alcohol-exposed children were found to be more variable and less accurate on tasks requiring motor timing and accuracy; also visual recognition of shape and color. Disruptions in motor timing behaviors that are dependent on sensory motor integration or motor execution, are indicative of cerebellar or basal ganglia damage (Wass, Simmons, Thomas, and Riley 2002). Slower reaction time suggests possible impairments in detection of a stimulus, stimulus discrimination, and motor planning time. Intellectual performance alone does not account for the deficits seen in visual and auditory attention;

and problems with auditory attention, particularly of omission, persist into adulthood (Connor, Streissguth, Sampson, Bookstein, and Barr 1999).

Neurocognitive impairments can be in all domains: attention, language, nonverbal learning, visual-motor integration, and the motor functions of fine-motor speed and coordination (Korkman, Kettunen, and Autti-Ramo 2003; Mattson, Riley, Gramling, Delis, and Jones 1998). In addition, Korkman and colleagues found the poorest performance on tests with attention and short-term working memory demands. Riley and colleagues (2003) found impairment of language, attention, and executive functions significant for all ages.

Offspring with no visible facial dysmorphy, have been found to have the same psychological problems in adulthood as those diagnosed with FAS (Lemoine 2003). All along the continuum from severe to mild impairment, children with FASD exhibit problem behaviors, such as alcohol and drug use, hyperactivity, impulsivity, poor socialization and communication skills (Mattson, Schoenfeld, and Riley 2001). Adaptive functioning for individuals with FASD, measured on the Vineland Adaptive Behavior Scale (VABS) and based on domains of communication, daily living, and socialization skills, is usually found to be even more deficit than academic achievement scores (Streissguth and O'Malley 2000). Because deficits in executive functioning reflect more than IQ or facial features, Connor, Sampson, Bookstein, Barr, and Streissguth (2000) recommend including executive functioning tests in a clinical evaluation.

In addition to IQ and basic academic testing, Sterling Clarren, Olson, Clarren, and Astley (2000) recommend two additional tests that provide information on verbal learning and memory, nonverbal memory, and visuospatial skills. The adult versions, of the California Verbal Learning Test and the Rey Complex Figure Test, for youngsters intelligent enough and old enough.

In a review of individual cases, Mattson and Riley (1998) found a mean intelligence quotient of 65, with a range of 20 to 120, for FAS. Evaluation of 415 patients found that only 24 percent with FAS and 7 percent with FAE have an IQ below the 70 IQ which has been used to qualify for special education services (Streissguth et al. 2004). Youngsters with learning and adaptive behavior problems commonly referred to as "falling through the cracks" remain a challenge for educators.

Barbara Page, a school psychologist, working in a small urban public school system for over 15 years, reports the few youngsters with FASD that have been qualified for service needed a medical diagnosis, qualifying under the handicapping condition "other health impaired." Youngsters who do not have a doctor's diagnosis, working below grade level, who may have FASD, youngsters with an IQ score in the mild to moderate range, are considered to be working up to their potential. Thus, not eligible for special education services. Undiagnosed students put educators at a disadvantage: is poor academic and poor social behavior caused by willfulness or organicity? Youngsters with FASD who are not mentally retarded, also need cognitive, adaptive, and social behavior interventions to function up to their potential.

The degree of cognitive disability in youngsters with FASD often goes unrecognized, this is especially true for those youngsters who look normal, whose intelligence is in the dull-normal range, and whose superficial behavior includes an air of alertness, appropriate affect, good superficial verbal skills, and a good sense of humor, characteristics that disguise their compromised cognitive functioning (Streissguth 1987). It is important that these children be referred for educational and clinical services.

Identification

Children prenatally exposed to alcohol can suffer from serious cognitive deficits in aspects of executive functioning critical for information processing and memory, that resulted from alcohol-related changes in brain neuroanatomy and chemistry. Disruption of neurodevelopmental processes, such as cell, migration, proliferation, differentiation, in addition to deterioration of neurons. Prenatal alcohol exposure produces a neuroanatomical pattern of incomplete or arrested development of the brain with disproportionate effects on the growth of specific tissues and brain structures. Archibald and colleagues (2001) found white matter volume (tracts of connections uniting one brain cell with another), more affected than gray matter volume (brain cells), in the cerebrum. Brain imaging studies have identified structural changes in various brain regions of individuals with FASD that may account for cognitive deficits.

Working memory incorporates the executive cognitive functions of acquiring, processing, and responding to information. The smaller caudate nucleus, part of the prefrontal circuit, which is involved with aspects of executive functioning, likely contributed to the fluency impairments in both verbal and nonverbal tasks found by Schonfeld, Mattson, Lang, Delis, and Riley (2001). Limitations in nonverbal fluency when creating distinct line designs, shifting between subtle differences in dots, and verbal fluency when shifting between differences in semantic categories (Schonfeld et al. 2001).

The lack of judgment resulting from cognitive impairments in abstract reasoning, executive functions, and memory impact academic, social, and basic daily living skills: poor judgment and failure to consider consequences are often described in the population with FASD (Connor et al. 2000). A poor memory may be compensated for by lying, filling in memory gaps with inappropriate inaccurate words, confabulation. The demands student's with FASD present to teachers, service providers, family, and other caregivers can be unrelenting.

Youngsters with FASD lack the ability to generalize, to use information from one situation and apply it to other similar situations. To understand what something means in a particular situation. Everything is in the present tense. Everything is a new task to youngsters who lack the ability to generalize. These youngsters have difficulty estimating consequences and learning from their mistakes. To complicate the picture further, their performance is often inconsistent and unpredictable, they *sporadically* master skills.

Comorbid

In addition to brain imaging information for diagnosis, Burd, Klug, Martsolf, and Kerbeshian (2003) found multiple comorbid mental disorders: attention deficit hyperactivity disorder, learning disabilities, mental retardation, speech and language disorders, mood disorders, oppositional defiant disorders, and self-injurious behaviors. "Thus, we may need to consider dysmorphia as markers that correlate with neuropsychiatric abnormalities and influence severity rather than a finding that defines them etiologically" (Burd et al. 2003). Burd advises that keeping facial dysmorphia as the essential diagnostic feature does not recognize the concept of a continuum of impairment with a neurobehavioral focus.

Secondary disabilities: Five adverse life outcomes were found in children, adolescents, and adults who had a diagnosis within the severity continuum of FASD (Streissguth et al. 2004). First, inappropriate sexual behaviors (ISB): such as, exposing, inappropriate touching, promiscuity, inappropriate sexual advances, were found across the individuals lifespan, increasing slightly with age. Second, disrupted school experience (DSE), which included suspensions, expulsions, and dropping out. The most frequent learning problems were attention problems and incomplete schoolwork, also repeatedly being disruptive in class. Third, was trouble with the law (TWL), including crimes against persons, shoplifting/theft, assault, burglary, and domestic violence. Fourth, confinement (CNF), including incarcerations and psychiatric hospitalizations. Fifth, alcohol and drug problems (ADP),

Table 4. Characteristics of Fetal Alcohol Spectrum Disorder

A. Premature birth
B. Prenatal and postnatal growth retardation
C. Cranial/facial abnormalities
D. Cardiovascular abnormalities
E. Renal abnormalities
F. Respiratory dysfunction
G. Cardiovascular abnormalities
H. Immune system dysfunction
I. Skeletal abnormalities
J. Central nervous system dysfunction
K. Neurological problems
    1. mental retardation
    2. disorganized play
    3. speech and language disorders
    4. learning disability
    5. decreased attention span
    6. tremulousness
    7. weak grasp
    8. clumsiness
    9. poor eye contact
    10. poor eye-hand coordination
    11. head and body rocking
    12. sleep disturbances
    13. visual impairment
    14. hearing impairment
    15. behavior
        a) insecure attachment patterns
        b) irritability in infancy
        c) hyperactivity in childhood
        d) conduct disorder in adolescence

(Abel 1984; Jones and Smith 1973; Streissguth et al. 1989)

including abuse of alcohol and street drugs. Good stable families were found to be a critical protective factor. "In other words, the smaller the percent of life that patients with FAS or FAE spent in stable/nurturing homes, the greater the risk that these patients as adolescents and adults would have more ISB, DSE, ADP, and TWL" (Streissguth et al. 2004).

Characteristics of FASD can be part of other syndromes or have causes other than maternal drinking. All youngsters with a flat philtrum or thin upper lip do not have FASD. For example, Hanley (2002) notes that other toxins which are known to put fetuses at risk for microcephaly are not included in studies of FASD.

Although FASD facial characteristics may fade a bit as youngsters mature, deficits persist throughout a lifespan and cannot be cured, no amount of good nutrition and postnatal care can erase the growth retardation and brain damage, the goal is management.

COCAINE

Cocaine is obtained from the leaves of *Erythroxylon coca* trees indigenous to South America where it has been used for centuries to increase endurance and reduce hunger. In the United States, the soft drink Coca Cola® was first made from cocaine using an extract of coca leaves and caffeine-rich kola beans. Coca has been used for over a millennium (Johanson and Fischman 1989).

In the 1800s, advances in chemistry isolated cocaine and morphine. Previously only available in natural form, by chewing leaves for example, a drug's impact was diluted. Remember stories of medicine men in wagons traveling across America selling tonics? "Heroin cough syrup was one of many pharmaceuticals at the turn of the century that contained mood-altering substances. The name 'heroin' was coined by Bayer in 1898, a year before the company introduced aspirin" (Musto 1991).

During the nineteenth century in American history opiates and cocaine were considered helpful compounds. "Benjamin Franklin regularly took laudanum—opium in alcohol extract—to alleviate the pain of kidney stones during the last few years of his life" (Musto 1991). After using these drugs, public concern with the negative consequences developed, resulting in the Harrison Act of 1914, which permitted the sale of cocaine only through prescriptions, and restricted

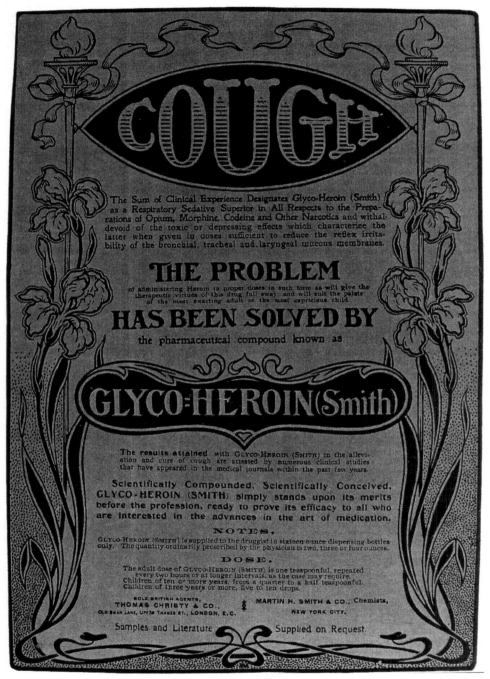

Figure 6. Drug Use History: Medicine Label. (Courtesy of *Scientific American*, July 1991, p. 41.)

habit-forming drugs to small amounts in nonprescription remedies.

The desirable affects of using cocaine are euphoric feelings of high energy and self-esteem. Within hours after use though, feelings of euphoria are replaced with anxiety, exhaustion, and depressive feelings (Singer, Garber, and Kliegman 1991). Substance abusing mothers may primarily use cocaine, yet they are likely to be polydrug users, using whatever drugs are available. In one study, Bozarth and Wise (1985) found that rats who self-administered unlimited supplies of cocaine developed exisodic patterns of excessive intake (binging). Their grooming behavior diminished, their general health deteriorated sharply, they lost 20 to 49 percent of their pretest body weight, and 90 percent were dead after 30 days. Extrapolating rat behavior to the human population may seem a reach, yet we see thin unkept mothers in poor general health that are taking cocaine. As recently as 1980, medical literature considered cocaine incapable of producing dependence (Gawin 1991).

COCAINE/POLYDRUG EFFECTS ON THE FETUS: RESEARCH

The negative complications of cocaine use during pregnancy were reported in 1983 when Acker and colleagues described the association between cocaine use and *abruptio placentae*, separation of the placenta from the uterine wall (Acker, Sachs, Tracey, and Wise 1983). Mothers are at risk for increased obstetrical complications: stillbirth, abruptio placentae, premature labor and delivery. The first report describing the effects of cocaine on neonatal outcome was published in 1985 (Chasnoff, Burns, Schnoll, and Burns 1985). Early research is filled with contradictions because of methodologic limitations; today the question remains whether effects on the offspring are transient or will persist.

"In the early years of our research we hypothesized that mechanical insults via intrauterine hypoxia served as the basis for the difficulties exhibited by the cocaine-exposed infant. That hypothesis clearly does not address the larger picture, however, for it appears that the impact of prenatal cocaine exposure is more subtle an insult, occurring at the level of the neurotransmitters and perhaps affecting the organization of neuronal transmission from subcortical regions of higher cortical control areas" (Chasnoff et al. 1998).

In human studies, the effects of cocaine can be separated only statistically from other drugs. Most studies use a combination of maternal interview, along with a newborn biological assessments of meconium and urine. Yet, there are methodological limitations in published medical studies on cocaine exposure, studies that failed to control for relevant variables: limited comparison groups, insufficient measurement of exposure, nonblind examinations, and behavioral outcome measures without quality of life relevance.

Because cocaine is often used in addition to a variety of other drugs, tobacco, alcohol, marijuana, heroin, methadone, the focus of this research section covers maternal polydrug use with cocaine as the primary drug, the addicted mother's drug of choice. Yet, despite the control of confounding variables for other drug use, with statistical analysis, effects of multiple drug use may be undercontrolled. Performance of the infants and toddlers studied can also be effected by passive intoxication from breast milk when nursing, in addition to inhaling ambient marijuana, cocaine, amphetamine, and tobacco smoke. Concerns of educators and other service providers are that studies on the cognitive development and behavior of infants prenatally exposed to cocaine/polydrugs do not go beyond seven to ten years of age; hence, providing insufficient information on the population of youngsters they are working with.

Neuroanatomical and neurochemical aberrations can result in loss of function and/or disorganization of brain activity. "Thus, cocaine-exposed infants appear to be at risk for later learning and behavioral disabilities from a biological perspective" (Singer, Farkas, and Kliegman 1992). The brain goes through a period of maturation; thus, one can't predict at an earlier age what deficits will show up as skills emerge. "The manifestations of negative effects of intrauterine drug exposure on infant development may become evident as these children get older and are required to engage in increasingly complex forms of thinking" (Chasnoff, Griffith, Freier, and Murray 1992). Increasing cognitive demands and social expectations may reveal previously unseen exposure effects. The question remains unanswered, does cocaine damage areas of the brain that do not exhibit impairment until school age, until adolescence?

What actions of cocaine are causing fetal damage: hypoxemia, the direct effects of the drug, and/or the drug's metabolic byproducts? Cocaine is a stimulant to the central nervous system, causing rapid heartbeat and constriction of arteries leading to the womb. Drug-induced alterations in placental blood flow may also effect the passage of nutrients to and wastes from the fetus.

What is known regarding cocaine's teratogenic actions on the fetus includes one or both of the following. First, reduced oxygen to the fetus from vasoconstriction can cause damage to developing structures or destruction of structures that previously have formed normally (Woods, Plessinger, and Clark 1987; Jones 1991; Viscarello, Ferguson, Nores, and Hobbins 1992). Second, direct cocaine toxicity: a rise in circulating cocaine metabolites and the hormone norepinephrine causing fetal vasoconstriction and exaggerated fetal cardiovascular responses. Fetal stroke can occur while in the womb or shortly after birth (Lange et al. 1989). "Women exposed to cocaine early in their pregnancies may be more at risk of teratogenic effects, while women exposed closer to delivery may be at increased risk of sudden cardio-vascular or cerebrovascular events" (Handler, Kistin, Davis, and Ferre 1991).

Cocaine causes dopamine and norepinephrine, chemical neuro-transmitters that transmit information between neurons, to remain longer in the neurons synaptic cleft, these neurotransmitters just keep firing, producing the cocaine "high." Cocaine prevents the reuptake of dopamine and norepinephrine; thus, greater concentrations circulate (Chasnoff 1991). Increased levels of norepinephrine in the first days of life may result in an elevated sympathetic tone (primarily the involun-tary muscles, a large part of the autonomic nervous system), with the stress of chronic hypoxemia resulting in a persistent increase in cate-cholamine release (a chemical that effects the nervous and cardiac sys-tems) (Mirochnick et al. 1997).

Alterations of neurotransmitters in the fetal central nervous system may disrupt the developing regulation of fetal behavioral states, influ-encing behavior in the newborn (Chasnoff and Griffith 1989; Tabor, Soffici, Smith-Wallace, and Yonekura 1991). According to Volpe (1992) "The neural systems most likely to be affected by cocaine are involved in neurologic and behavioral functions (attention, arousal, motivation and social interaction, for example) . . ."

Starting at 32 weeks, intrauterine neurobehavior testing can be done using sound. When you startle the fetus with a sudden noise, the normal fetus will have a rapid rise in heart rate, kick around; then slow down, find its fist to self comfort, and then calm down. The cocaine-exposed fetus jumps, cannot calm down and his/her heart rate stays elevated for hours. Even in the womb, these babies respond abnormally to stimulation. Hyperaroused, cocaine effected babies have difficulty shutting out and organizing information (Chasnoff 1987).

Susan Stanley in *Maternity Ward* (1992) based her book on the evening shift in the labor and delivery department at the Oregon Health Sciences University Hospital in Portland, and captures the ramifications of maternal crack use on the fetus. "One time a woman came into the prep room. She was using IV crack on a frequent basis. Karen gave her an ultrasound and saw that the baby was turning somersaults in the uterus. Literally. Right there on the screen, like on a television set, you could see the limbs jerking and kicking, the baby shifting from being all over on the left side of the woman's abdomen to being on the right side. That baby was so stimulated by the crack that it would change from breech to vertex several times in the space of a few minutes."

WITHDRAWAL

At delivery, drug transfer ceases, but drug metabolism continues along with a cycle of excretion and reabsorption lasting for days or weeks, possibly, leaving the infant in withdrawal. This baby remains irritable for six to eight weeks and doesn't respond well to its environment for two or three months. Milder forms of withdrawal persist for four to six months. Withdrawal problems involve autonomic nervous system instability: the involuntary regulation of digestion, respiration, circulation. A baby in the biological/neurological recovery of withdrawal has: high respiratory and heart rates, increased tremulousness and startles, irregular sleeping, high-pitched cry, fever, sweating, seizures, voracious sucking (sucking on fists), jitteriness and excessive muscle tone, including *hypotonic* (floppy), and *hypertonic* (extreme muscle tension, overextending, stiff). Easily overstimulated, overloaded by environmental stimuli, these babies' withdraw into sleep or crying (Schneider and Chasnoff 1992).

CHARACTERISTICS OF FETAL COCAINE/POLYDRUG
EXPOSURE (FDE)

Eyler and colleagues (2001) found that early effects of prenatal cocaine exposure stand alone, appearing not to be related to withdrawal. While children with FASD commonly have identifying facial and other physical abnormalities, children prenatally exposed to cocaine have few physical manifestations. The bulk of evidence on prenatal cocaine exposure finds a greater percentage of neurologic damage than motor deficits or poor growth patterns (Burkett et al. 1990). What is unknown is the extent of risk and the reversibility of the injury (Gingras, et al. 1992; Nordstrom-Klee, Delaney-Black, Covington, Ager, & Sokol 2002). Long-term effects are unknown, most studies cover the age range from birth to age three, a few more follow offspring to age seven. Thus, it is unknown if damage persists into childhood and adulthood; or what secondary disabilities could result.

Frank, Augustyn, Knight, Pell, and Zuckerman (2001) reviewed thirty-six studies, and found the data not convincing that in utero exposure to cocaine was the causal factor for adverse developmental consequences in children up to age six. Multiple other risk factors, found in the population of substance using adults, correlated with negative cognitive and behavioral outcomes (Frank et al. 2001).

Behaviors of serious concern are: decreased interactive behavior, a low threshold for frustration, decreased consolability, less adequate ability to regulate states of consciousness, agitated sleep, and poor feeding. These concerns may be caused by, or exacerbated by, poor parent-infant interaction; inadequate stimulation gives the brain little to learn from.

When reviewing research on the outcome of infants exposed prenatally to cocaine, the following physical defects found included: lower birth weights, shorter lengths, smaller head circumferences, skull and skeletal bone defects, eye defects, genitourinary tract malformations, anomalies of the kidneys, respiratory abnormalities, cardiac arrhythmias and central nervous system deficits (Gingras et al. 1992; Chasnoff et al. 1985). Inferior visual and auditory-orienting skills have been found in infants prenatally cocaine-exposed. The fetus is also at risk for intrauterine growth retardation resulting in reduction in birth weight and length (Nordstrom-Klee, et al. 2002). Also, cardiac *arrhythmias* (heart rhythm disturbance), coronary artery spasm, myocardial and cerebral *infarctions* (dead tissue deprived of blood supply), strokes, seizures, and sudden deaths (Burkett et al. 1990; Singer et al. 1992; Gingras et al. 1992). When reacting to reduced oxygen, the fetus directs blood to the brain away from the extremities. Limb defects result from this lack of blood: missing toes, fingers, an arm or leg (Hoyme et al. 1990).

Bada and colleagues (2002) found the following central nervous system (CNS) signs to be highly associated with prenatal exposure to cocaine or cocaine and opiates: jitteriness/tremors, irritability, hypertonia, a high-pitched cry, and infants that are difficult to console.

Prenatal exposure to cocaine has not been found to be related to a global IQ measure of cognitive development. Based on rat brain studies, cognitive deficits appear to be related to slower acquisition rather than an inability to learn (Dow-Edwards, Freed, Fico 1990). Using animal models, Gendle, and colleagues (2004), found subtle impairments related to regulation in the domains of attention, arousal, and response to stress. Significant permanent effects on the structure and form of the cortical outer layers of the brain, were found in mice with fetal cocaine exposure: a reduction in the number of cells, inappropriate positioning of neurons, and altered glial morphology (Kosofsky and Wilkins 1998). Mayes (2003) found in a review of the research, animal models parallel reports from cocaine-exposed preschool and schoolaged children, who had deficits in selective attention and in information processing. These deficits in animal subjects reflect processes of learning and memory especially crucial to situations that demand attention to less obvious but relevant stimuli, when more conspicuous, but not necessarily relevant stimuli occur in the same context. This looks like the student who seldom gets the point in a lively classroom. Yet, some research on human subjects with prenatal cocaine exposure find intellectual and behavioral problems low or nonexistent (Bennett, Bendersky and Lewis 2002).

Language — limited expressive language; comprehension; localizing to sounds

Given that damage from teratogens can be subtle and not manifest for many years: standard language evaluation instruments may not find slight variations in the pragmatics, syntax, and semantics of language. Infants respond to their own names by four and a half months, by six months they respond appropriately to "mommy," by about seven and a half months they begin to distinguish words from fluent speech, and from about eight months, infants begin to attach meanings to words.

Delays in language development have been found in the first year of life for youngsters with FDE. Singer and colleagues (2001) found delays in auditory comprehension skills considered to be precursors of receptive language: localizing to sounds, visually following an object, attending to toys or books, and playing social games. Based on a global language assessment of children to age three years, prenatal cocaine exposure resulted in an average of 15 percent of a standard deviation (SD), lower performance (Morrow et al. 2003). Following children to age seven years, Bandstra and colleagues (2002) found a 1/5 SD in total language function for children with prenatal cocaine exposure. Delaney-Black and colleagues (2000), found six-year-old children who were prenatally exposed to cocaine were 2.4 times more likely to be in the low language ability group: showing less expressive language vocabulary diversity (fewer number of word types per number of words spoken). Children evaluated at four years of age who were exposed to cocaine in utero, lagged behind in basic language skills: semantics, syntax, and the order in which words are put together to make phrases and sentences (Lewis, et al. 2004).

Sensitivity

Lester and colleagues (2003) looked at infant auditory brain responses at one month, finding effects were more pronounced at lower, rather than higher intensities. Indicating the possibility of hypersensitivity, these infants require a lower intensity stimulus.

Impairments in neurobehavioral performance, particularly for the regulation of arousal, were found at 3 weeks (Tronick, Frank, Cabral, Mirochnick, and Zuckerman 1996). Infants and preschool-aged children exposed gestationally to cocaine exhibit a lower threshold for stress when exposed to novel challenges; thus, are likely less able to deal with stressful conditions. They require more stimulation to reach optimal states of arousal but modulate higher states of arousal less well and, therefore, often quickly become overaroused (Mayes, Domenic, Suddhasatta, and Heping 2003).

Medical foster moms' describe having cared for cocaine addicted infants with thresholds for sensory stimulation so low they dislike being touched, who act like their skin hurts. Infants who cry when they have a bath, the water hurts. Even the touch of clothing hurts them, the fewer clothes they have on the less fussy they are. Many parents *or shoes* report their children have problems getting dressed and keeping their clothes on, that youngsters don't outgrow this. They found firm pressure, rather than a gentle touch, is less disturbing to this child with tactile defensiveness.

Hypersensitive newborns may have to be put on pillows before rocking them. "The less I held him the better he was," a mother described finding it a challenge to provide stimulation at a level below the infant's threshold. Baby massage had to be done in a dark room to reduce the stimulation. Focused stimulation helps this infant avoid the overstimulation that results from the difficulty of tuning out irrelevant stimuli. The infant must develop enough control over the ability to receive and shut out stimuli to accept the stimulation necessary for development, self-regulation, and organization.

Intellectual Functioning

Using the Bayley Mental and Motor Scales of Infant Development scores at two years, prenatally cocaine-exposed children were twice as likely as controls to have significant cognitive delays throughout the first two years of life. Because these scores are predictive of later cognitive outcomes, the children may continue to have learning problems (Singer, Arendt, et al. 2002). Again at three years of age, lower Bayley mental performance scores were found for offspring prenatally exposed to cocaine (Mayes, et al. 2003). Continuing to assess long-term cognitive effects of prenatal cocaine exposure, Singer and colleagues (2004) looked at IQ scores of four-year-olds. Results of the Wechsler Preschool and Primary Scales of Intelligence-Revised found small decrements on the subscales: visual-spatial skills, general knowledge, and arithmetic skills. Prenatal cocaine exposure was not related to a lower full-scale IQ, but was associated with a lower birth head circumference, and a lower likelihood of a full-scale IQ, above the normative mean, average of 100, at age four years (ibid).

Children age eight to nine years who had prenatal exposure to cocaine were as efficient at a visuospatial maze task, after repeated exposures. But, their slowed visuomotor speed and efficiency resulted in poorer performance involving memory functions that include sustained attention and information processing (Schroder, Snyder, Sielski, and Mayes 2004).

Motor Functioning

Infant developmental scales may underevaluate because they assess quantitative rather than qualitative aspects of motor development (Schneider, Lee, and Chasnoff 1988). Developmental tests are structured, favoring the strengths of children; whereas, these youngsters have deficits primarily in the quality of their responses: poorer motor abilities, poorer motor organization, and more abnormal reflexes. For instance, developmental scales for cocaine and polydrug effected newborns reflect unusual patterns of motor development; youngsters with excessive muscle tone who crawl early, walk early, and stand early (Chasnoff, Hatcher, and Burns 1982). The key to motor planning is a body perception with accurate tactile, proprioceptive, and vestibular information. An atypical motor development course was found in infants with compromised motor development at four and seven months, who had differences at one month or at 15 months. Fetters and Tronick (1996) speculate on these results; that there could be several different developmental pathways to the achievement of motor milestones, that the prerequisite subsystems may appear unevenly during development but consolidate within a normal developmental period for later achievement milestones. In clinic practice Fetters and Tronick see motor development problems no longer evident at seven months, yet, raise concerns that motor skills are fundamental to infant exploratory behavior; compromises in motor abilities can limit intellectual development.

The Neonatal Behavioral Assessment Scale (NBAS) measures infants' states of consciousness in response to environmental stimulation, "There are twenty-eight behavioral items. These assess the newborns capacity (1) to organize states of consciousness, (2) to habituate to disturbing events, (3) to attend to and process simple and, in some cases, complex environmental events, (4) to control motor tone and activity while attending to these events, and (5) to perform integrated motor acts, such as putting a hand in the mouth, maintaining the head upright while sitting . . ." (Brazelton and Cramer 1991). The NBAS identifies the positive characteristics of a difficult baby and provides a tool for understanding how the newborn handles stimulation. Thus, the parents' expectations can be framed, so they can respond appropriately to the baby's state of consciousness, and adjust their interactions to the newborn's behavior (Brazelton and Cramer 1991). Information from the NBAS can be used for intervention in potentially dysfunctional parent-infant interactions, before poor parenting patterns become well-established (Tedder 1991).

Looking at rhesus monkeys, prenatal cocaine exposure was capable of producing neurobehavioral deficits detectable by NBAS-like testing: significant neurobehavioral deficits were found for orientation, state control, motor maturity, and it was observed that less time was spent manipulating a toy (He, Bai, Champoux, Suomi, and Lidow 2004). They also found these deficits were detected only by the second or third week of life when the infant monkeys reached appropriate levels of development.

On the NBAS, newborns exposed to cocaine have lower scores on social interactions, the ability to maintain alertness, to use motor control, visual and hearing orientation, and their ability to organize and respond to environmental stimuli (Chasnoff et al. 1985). Chasnoff found many of the cocaine-exposed infants never reached an alert state at all during the NBAS exam. The ability to attend is dependent on the infant's state of consciousness. Infants who achieved alertness required adult control of external stimuli, so that they could focus on one specific stimulus. Most of the cocaine-exposed infants were capable of only fleeting attention to a given stimulus before displaying signs of distress. Responses to overstimulation included color changes, rapid breathing, irregular sleeping, high-pitched crying, disorganized motor activity, and frantic gaze aversion. Chasnoff found that each infant seemed to have a threshold for overstimulation, before moving into a state of sleeping or frenzied crying (Chasnoff 1989). Corwin and colleagues (1992) found "Infants exposed to cocaine produced fewer cry utterances, more short cries, and less crying in the hyperphonation mode. These findings suggest a pattern of underaroused neurobehavioral function." Eisen and colleagues (1991) assessed fifty-two newborns on the NBAS, the cocaine-exposed newborns demonstrated more stress behaviors and had less developed *habituation* skills. They were less able to decrease a response to a stimulus after repeated exposure, when the stimulus no longer require a response or was novel.

Caution: there is a danger of concluding that every youngster demonstrating a few characteristics has FASD or FDE. Many charac-

Table 5. Characteristics of the Cocaine/Polydrug-Effected Infant/Child.

A. Low birth weight
B. Strokes
C. Hypersensitivity
D. Rocking
E. Tactile defensiveness
F. Poor eye contact
G. Auditory Avoidance
H. Strokes
I. Seizures
J. Disorders of alertness
K. Respiratory dysfunction
L. Cardiovascular abnormalities
M. Delayed language development
N. Difficulty organizing information
O. Flat or irritable behavior
P. Low scores on the Brazelton Neonatal Behavioral Assessment Scale
    1. social interactions
    2. the ability to maintain alertness
    3. motor control
    4. visual and hearing orientation
    5. the ability to organize and respond to environmental stimuli
Q. Scales of Infant Motor Development
    1. excessive muscle tone
    2. abnormal posturing
    3. unusual and unpredictable course of development
       a) crawl early
       b) walk early
       c) stand early
R. Drug withdrawal
    1. Irritable for six to eight weeks
    2. Milder forms of withdrawal persist for 4 to 6 months
    3. High respiratory and heart rates
    4. Increased tremulousness and startles
    5. Irregular sleeping
    6. High-pitched cry
    7. Fever
    8. Sweating
    9. Seizures
    10. Voracious sucking
    11. Deficient in the ability to respond to the human face and voice
    12. Demanding, yet inconsolable
    13. Difficulties interacting with others
    14. Difficulty coping with an unstructured environment

Source: Chasnoff et al. 1982; Chasnoff et al. 1986; Chasnoff et al. 1992; Schneider and Chasnoff 1987; Gingras et al. 1992.

teristics are shared with other disorders. Educators must weigh research inconsistences with the individual differences their students demonstrate when pinpointing deficits to be circumvented and delays to be remediated.

Chapter 3

BEHAVIOR

Up to now we have looked at the physical and intellectual characteristics of youngsters with FASD and then at youngsters with
FDE. In this chapter behavioral characteristics are described in light
of social implications. The FASD child who wants to touch everyone,
the child with FDE, who has a low threshold to stimulation, who
avoids touch. Youngsters who's poor judgement is exacerbated
because they haven't developed empathy with others. Brain damage
from prenatal exposure to a teratogen can disrupt how brain systems
interact when creating and maintaining memories. Learned and genetically affected connections between brain cells, often accompanied by
the strong memory enhancement of emotional arousal, shape who we
are. The development of prosocial and moral reasoning is influenced
by the child's neurological ability to respond empathically and nonag-
gressively to emotion eliciting situations. This chapter is based on
medical, psychological, and educational research, highlighted with
interviews.

Altered physiological and behavioral reactions can influence social
functioning negatively, interfering with the development of behavior
patterns necessary for normal development. A challenge, for behavior
as well as academic skills, is the undiagnosed child who looks normal,
with neurobehavioral dysfunction, who is not recognized at an early
age to have special needs. The child with limited adaptability to stress
and ability to solve problems, the child with a limited emotional tone
and range of feelings, is ill-equipped to tackle the development and
maintenance of interpersonal relations.

Physiological effects of prenatal drug exposure extend into emotional development: affect regulation, development of social relation-

ships, using social cues to make interpersonal judgments, and cognitive development in functional and symbolic aspects, beginning with children's play.

> Clearly, the changes in social behavior observed in adults with FAS could be a function of many things including their genetic background, alcohol-induced alterations in brain structures involved in social behavior, abnormal childhood socialization processes, and abnormalities in social learning processes throughout the lifespan. (Kelly, Day, and Streissguth 2000)

Nancy Jones, Field, Davalos, and Hart (2004) found in children aged three to six years, prenatally exposed to cocaine, nonemphatic behavior correlated with electrical activity in the right frontal cortex. A greater right frontal EEG asymmetry and a greater overall EEG activation, was found in both the right and left hemispheres. This brain activity pattern suggests these youngsters may have higher intensity responses even during nonstressful conditions, possibly compromising their ability to finish a task. Other studies support this, suggesting cocaine-exposed children are more temperamentally difficult, and hypersensitive. These individual differences in emotional responses, effect caregiver-infant relationships. Mothers of cocaine-exposed youngsters were found to be less likely to express approval statements, less able to tune into the child's temperament (Jones et al. 2004).

BEHAVIORS OF CONCERN

Common concerns for behavior are: lack of motivation, no patience, immaturity, hyperactivity, impulsiveness, lack of inhibition, staying on task, distracting others, and dealing with change. In many cases the range and extent of behavioral deficits demand extensive supervision and attention. The impact of hyperactivity is exacerbated by the lack of impulse control, poor memory, and poor judgment. Socially, the child with FASD is easily influenced, lacking the judgment to respond to abstract social rules. Many are "touchy," resulting in inappropriate social behavior. They don't read social cues, they stand too close, they touch and hug everyone. Maladaptive behaviors of adolescents with FASD include lying, distractibility, poor judgment, defiance, and impulsivity. These behaviors threaten vocational success, social opportunities, and independent adult living (Streissguth et al. 1991).

Steinhausen and colleagues looked at children with FASD for behavioral phenotype characteristics based on either biology, heredity or environment. Behaviors they found were: communication disturbances, disruptive, self-absorbed, anxious, antisocial, and autistic. Intelligence and gender were not correlated with behavior, also youngsters with a diagnosis of FAS did not have more problems with behavior than youngsters with mild expressions of FASD (Steinhausen, Willms, Metzke, and Spohr, 2003). Problems with behavior are seen across all degrees of damage severity. Parent ratings of behavior on the Achenbach Child Behavior Checklist revealed significant concerns regarding behavioral disturbances in all youngsters with FASD not related to facial dysmorphology, intellectual functioning, or socioeconomic status (Mattson and Riley 2000). Again, irrespective of severity of FASD the Vineland Adaptive Behavior Scale revealed deficits in adaptive functioning in three domains: communication, daily living skills, and socialization. In addition, declines in socialization became more significant with age (Whaley, O'Connor, and Gunderson 2001). O'Connor and colleagues found children with FASD are at high risk for major psychiatric disorders: significantly 61 percent met criteria for a diagnosis of mood disorder (O'Connor, et al 2002). In addition to the mood disorder depression, Famy, Streissguth, and Unis (1998) found a high incidence of alcohol or drug dependence. Baumbach (2002) also found that 49 percent of adolescents and adults with FASD displayed inappropriate sexual behavior. Looking at treatment, Baumbach recommends expectations for behavioral self-control be reasonable: based on frustration tolerance and delay of gratification in the real world.

Attention Deficits

If you are not paying attention to social information how can you develop social skills? Based on studies of brain structures using magnetic resonance imaging (MRI), researchers have found that significant differences exist in the corpus callosum (fibers connecting the right and left brain hemispheres) of children with attention deficit-hyperactivity disorder (ADHD) (Hynd et al. 1991). Youngsters with attention deficits often display a short attention span, restlessness, poor concentration, and general distractibility. In classrooms some youngsters appear to have attention spans of only a few seconds, so short they may not have sufficient time to focus their attention. Youngsters with FASD/FDE demonstrate many of the same behaviors found in children with ADHD. Nanson and Hiscock (1990) compared attention and behavior problems in 20 children who have FAS/FAE with 20 children who have attention deficit disorder (ADD) and 20 normal controls. Their results suggest ". . . although children with FAS/FAE are significantly more impaired intellectually than are children with classical ADD, the attentional problems of both groups of children are similar" (Nanson and Hiscock 1990). Both groups of children had difficulty maintaining attention and inhibiting impulsive responses. How this impacts academic and social learning is that once attention is successfully focused, the poor memory of individuals with FASD require information to be repeated over and over.

Table 6. Behavioral Characteristics: FASD/FDE

- Behavioral extremes
- No motivation
- No patience
- Immaturity
- Lack of affect
- Lethargy
- Hyperactivity
- Lack of impulse control
- Preoccupation with objects
- Preservative behavior
- Apparent lack of fear
- Show no remorse
- Decreased task persistence
- Distractibility: self and others
- Dealing with change: inflexible
- Regressive behavior
- Ritualized behaviors
- Aggressive behaviors
- Oppositional behaviors
- Self abuse
- Self stimulation
- Decreased pro-social behaviors
- Poor social judgment
- Lack empathy for others
- Insecure attachment patterns
- Avoid touch
- Clinging, "touchy"

Hyperactivity - Sluggishness

Some hyperactivity may be related to brain stem deficits in arousal. Cocaine alters the metabolism of the neurotransmitter norepinephrine, which is important in brain functions regulating arousal (Gingras, O'Donnell, and Hume 1990). A state of sensory deprivation results if the brain stem reticular system is not producing sufficient arousal or letting through enough stimuli to maintain arousal, the child is "underaroused" (Reynolds 1981). We can all relate to becoming disorganized when we are sleepy or fatigued. Drugs like methylphenidate (Ritalin) raise arousal levels, thereby allowing a child to reduce the activity level needed to alleviate an aversive state of sensory depravation. When the child is overaroused the reticular system may be failing to screen stimuli. In a youngster with brain stem deficits in arousal, excessive stimulation or insufficient stimulation may cause the same hyperactive behavior. The youngster is working to establish a comfortable level of arousal.

The negative aspects of hyperactivity are intensified by the lack of impulse control, poor memory, and poor judgment that result from damage to the limbic system which is involved in the behavioral and emotional expression of eating, fighting, fleeing, and sexual behavior. In addition, the hippocampus of the limbic system, is involved in learning and memory processing.

MENTAL HEALTH THERAPY

A good place for assessment and treatment by mental health professionals to start is taking an adequate history, including maternal drinking and drug use during pregnancy. Recognizing an organic basis for behavior/learning problems can direct treatment to *educational* rather than insight-based cognitive behavioral therapies or medication interventions. Identification of the specific functional problem can guide educationally based therapies to improve behavioral management of social interactions.

> Recognizing an organic basis for behavior/learning problems, can direct treatment to educational rather than insight-

based cognitive behavioral therapies or
medication intervention.

Giancola, Shoal, and Mezzich (2001) looked at the involvement of
executive functioning with substance use disorder, in adolescents.
They speculate that limited executive functioning made cognitive regulation of behavior ineffectual, finding antisocial behavior was significantly related to drug use. Continuing to look at behavior, Giancola
and Mezzich (2003) found a difficult temperament: ". . . the susceptibility to become easily and intensely emotionally distressed, the inability to sooth or calm oneself after experiencing such distress, the inability to stop ruminating about a particular problem, as well as the inability to regulate strong thrill-seeking or high irritability levels . . ." important risk factors in drug use. Impaired cognitive regulation of behavior, abstract reasoning, and attentional skills compromise the ability to
understand social cues, to understand the potentially negative consequences of engaging in high-risk behaviors. Deficiencies in cognitive
skills can also lead to misattributions in the perception of threat or hostility in conflict situations, and interfere with the ability to execute a
series of responses in the proper order and manner, to avoid potentially volatile social interactions and dangerous situations. Use of a
practical strategy in response to this, Doris Rademacher-Dramov, a
high school teacher, keeps a list of hostility-taming phrases such as
"can you help me?" to remind herself of what she could be saying. She
distracts the student from the behavior that elicited the misinterpreta-
tion, and rewards the student's change to more appropriate interactions: strategies for the behavior monitoring child-bearing aged adolescents need.

Streissguth and O'Malley (2000) note several factors affecting treatment by mental health professionals. That FASD is a chronic neuropsychiatric condition usually not considered in the differential diagnosis of mental disorders. That the Diagnostic and Statistical Manual
of Mental Disorders (DSM-IV) does not have a way ". . . to understand
the complex interplay of biological and social influences in the development of children . . ." with FASD (ibid), and thus integrate existing
knowledge in the development of treatment protocols. Streissguth and
O'Malley would like to see a treatment protocol; steps to be taken,
based on an understanding of how biology influences the development of children with FASD.

Learning social behavioral responses and learning academic skills use the same neurological processes: connections in the brain are changed. This is why a productive mental health therapy protocol combines medication with behavioral/teaching approaches to learn successful ways of thinking and acting. Although treatment for individuals with FASD often include medication, research on medication treatment is scarce. Parents I have interviewed have not found medication successful. Yet, the subset of children with FASD and coexisting ADHD, may have aspects of ADHD responsive to medication.

Estenson (2003), writing in the FASD newsletter *Iceberg*, recommends use of a "life coach" to help adults develop a successful social life, because adults with FASD often misread the intentions and reactions of others. The focus is on real-life norms. A "life coach" can be more therapeutic than sympathetic: helping the person organize their thoughts before expressing them, modeling interpersonal behavior, advising when to use replacement behaviors, and assisting with the activities of everyday life.

Addiction

Maternal recovery from addiction is a major step in the successful development of children prenatally exposed to drugs/alcohol, who remain with their biological parents. For the parents who have cognitive deficits: impaired problem-solving skills or attention deficits, Jerry Annand's treatment recommendations may be successful. Annand (2002) suggests the mental health addiction recovery treatment model using cognition to achieve understanding and insight, be replaced with a focus on behavior, for persons with cognitive disabilities. "The shift must be from cognition to behavior." Development of treatment goals to support *routines of living*, based on the AA saying "You can't think your way to sober acting, but you can act your way to sober thinking." Annand suggests turning the twelve steps of AA into action statements, what can the person *do*.

Replace cognitive-based insight with problem-solving tools. If you change the conditions the child is in, then you change the kind of behavior elicited. Use replacement behaviors: replace unsuccessful behaviors with ones that are personally relevant, behaviors that match the individual's strengths and that fit the demands of a situation.

Baer, Sampson, Barr, Connor, and Streissguth (2003) followed offspring for 21 years and found prenatal alcohol exposure to be a risk factor for the development of negative consequences related to alcohol use: passing out, blackouts, and being physically sick. Temperament influences the management of drinking activities: responding impulsively, making especially risky choices before, during, or after drinking heavily.

EMOTIONAL EXPRESSION

Prenatal damage can involve portions of the brain responsible for emotional expression. From birth these youngsters break into the overly affectionate touchy, clinging FASD youngster; or the cocaine/polydrug effected noncuddler, overly sensitive to stimuli, that resists touch, seldom laughs or smiles. They may fail to understand affective states, unable to grasp emotionally their or other's behavior. Importantly their emotional response style influences the amount of sensory stimulation others provide them. We expect children to be physically and mentally active, to spontaneously initiate experiences. We delight in their exploration. Many drug/alcohol effected youngsters show us little of this natural curiosity. A thread of behavioral consistency is often missing. Extremes of behavior are common; from apathy to aggression, passivity to hyperactivity, indiscriminate trust to extreme suspicion. Bizarre reactions to normal sensory stimulation, noise, pain, touch, and smell follow youngsters that had low thresholds for sensory stimulation as infants. Some youngsters self abuse: hit, bite, pick at, and pinch themselves. They may engage in self-stimulation such as repetitive touching or moving of a body part, flapping hands. They may engage in ritualistic behavior; such as, washing hands repeatedly, touching the edges of a desk before beginning work, or lining up pencils in a box. Youngsters may have preservative behavior, repeating the same thing over and over. Rather than using adults for approval, comfort, securing objects, or play, behavior with adults may be clingy.

Youngsters may have poor inner controls, giggles turn into screams, spontaneous temper tantrums, with no apparent cause, or overreacting to "no." With aggressive behavior: fighting, kicking, pinching, biting, pushing, pulling hair, spitting, and throwing. Youngsters who demonstrate oppositional behavior are resistant to adult directions showing dislike and hostility. It looks callous when they show no remorse for wrongdoing, denying everything, even when standing in the midst of proof. Youngsters may not express fear, grief, worry or show concern for hurt peers.

Failure

As individuals experience failure retrieving information from memory "I forgot–I can't remember," a negative emotional response is likely to accompany that failure. For example, long hesitations that accompany information retrieval when the youngster is upset, may be filled with a variety of unrelated information. It is also possible that an increased number of incorrect responses will be accompanied by the youngster's responding immediately with any kind of response, showing interest in other matters, or other unconstructive negative behaviors. Frustration with a task may exacerbate the physiological difficulty a youngster is having.

Foster moms have found many youngsters with FASD/FDE to be pack-rats, hoarders. They just grab something quickly and put it away in a secret place. "So fast, they are so fast." Watches, keys, pens, "you put it down, and its gone." Parents find they must lock up valuable items the child is attracted to.

Betty, a beautiful 13-year-old foster child, like many other youngsters with FAE , "never confesses to anything." She has no guilt, and gets mad because you don't believe her. Betty's mother reports, this seems like misbehavior, yet "there are just certain things she's drawn to." There may be damage to the portion of Betty's brain that initiates emotional expression. Youngsters with FASD/FDE have a limited range and variety of behavioral responses they can draw upon in a given situation. In addition, they lack the judgment to respond to abstract social rules. They can't predict what will happen as a result of their behavior. Thus, the response they choose may be inappropriate.

Inflexible, they may not be able to interrupt and redirect their own behavior. We, along with the child, are unable to predict what they will do next. Constant monitoring and attention may be needed. Youngsters with FDE are likely to require specific instruction in those prosocial skills which nondrug effected youngsters easily acquire by observing and interacting socially: using the appropriate social skills of stranger identification, social boundaries, and cooperative play.

SOCIAL BEHAVIOR

It looks like misbehavior when youngsters never seem to be disposed to or drawn to creative constructive behaviors; almost with a negative penchant toward unproductive patterns. Independent play, new behaviors, and exploration are often unconstructive; seemingly without purpose. How do we accept that this child has neurological damage that results in poor social judgment rather than a child with bad intent? That central nervous system defects may underlie behavioral deficits. The perceptual information a child with FASD/FDE is responding to may differ from what we are perceiving. Behavior is determined by how what is perceived is interpreted; the child may hold misperceptions about the way the world works. Hence, behaviors may be based on little if any understanding of the situation or event, or evaluation of the consequences.

Robin Lindsley, an early childhood development specialist, finds it important to realize that the youngster is damaged, that "he's not doing it on purpose," he can't help it. The child's behavioral aberrations come from brain defects related to maternal drug use. "He isn't bad, but I still can't cope with it," describes feelings other teachers have brought up. Robin recommends that teachers stop labeling the child or the behavior as bad, and decide to focus on attainable behavioral goals. Robin described Jim, a youngster with possible FDE, as a boy who couldn't track information. He couldn't screen out the irrelevant information that would enable him to focus on key information. Even when he was interested in the activity he would wander from place to place. During story time when the class was sitting on the rug, he would roll around on it. He couldn't complete anything. Realizing that Jim was damaged helped Robin accept the intent of his behavior and focus on help, rather than discipline. Given his skills and behavior, "What can I do to teach him in a busy classroom."

Even though children with mild FASD/FDE may look normal and may have good superficial skills, their disabilities can frustrate adults unfamiliar with their backgrounds. These youngsters violate your expectations. Some youngsters have deviant behaviors though average IQ scores. Some can appear normal, yet a seventeen-year-old can have the social, functional, and intellectual age of a seven-year-old. Youngsters may be attractive and have good verbal abilities, yet poor abstract thinking. They can't figure things out. Poor reasoning, inflexible, unable to adjust to a new demand or a change in activity. These students are often placed in higher academic situations than they can function in. Youngsters that look normal, with cognitive deficits trying very hard to pose as normal, mild FASD characteristics are likely to be masked by the time they reach adulthood. Youngsters with mild FASD that are normal looking are often misjudged because they tend to be talkative and outgoing. "No one dreams their nervous systems are impaired" (Steinmetz 1992).

A medical foster mom adopted a 13-year-old girl, Kim, with FDE, who needed medication to manage depression. It takes all Kim's energy just to act normal. Others expect more of her than she is capable of because she doesn't look handicapped; her disability isn't on the outside. Students made fun of Kim so much, she didn't want to continue going to school. FASD robbed her of a sense of social and intellectual competence.

Youngsters with FASD/FDE can have a sense of disconnectedness. Youngsters that are unable to predict the probability of an event occurring, who are unable to benefit from the incidental learning most of us use, may not integrate important subtleties of information; thus, may not be able to react to important abstract social rules. Their poor social judgment and impulsivity can result in negative peer interactions. Another medical foster mom has a seven-year-old boy with FAS. Children make fun of him, "he slaps the children, and then he gets in trouble." Youngsters with FASD/FDE may act hostile and aggressive: slapping, biting, kicking, and often showing no remorse. Difficulty with impulse control gets them into trouble and can develop into lying, cheating, stealing, and physically aggressive behaviors.

Behavior problems are often a result of information processing deficits. How much of their difficult, socially unacceptable behavior is the result of a sense of inferiority and inadequacy? How much is neurologically based? Distracted, they have difficulty concentrating, unable to perform routine activities routinely, they cannot continue after an interruption. Are they able to internalize moral rules and develop a conscience? Youngsters with FASD/FDE are impacted by the limitations they bring to learning social rules.

When their expectations exceed their capabilities, children are susceptible to a sense of inferiority or inadequacy that may seriously inhibit their ability to understand and perform. Beth Caruso's prekindergarten students find it harder to accept peers when its a social skill, rather than intellect that is missing. The students' forget about the handicap and think "he's mean." They find it hard to make friends with youngsters that have compromised social skills. Beth finds herself saying many times a day "I like you–I don't like what you're doing."

Teachers are concerned about the youngsters who have FASD/FDE, and who are unable to see another's point of view. Youngsters with poor social judgment who show no empathy with others and lack impulse control, present a scary picture. "How can you get along if you can't understand what others are feeling or thinking? What will they grow up to be like?" The internal scrutiny upon which to base responsible behavior is precarious when moral development is not based on empathy with others.

Self-awareness emerges at about two years, along with pronouns such as "me" and "mine." This sense of self is followed by the appearance of self-conscious emotions: empathy, jealousy, and embarrassment. Self-awareness is established by neurological and physical feedback connecting relevant social cognitive information. The body is aware of itself, through proprioception (sensory information from joints, muscles, and tendons), contributing to the social cognitive information the individual brings to a situation. A youngster with damage to these connections, like one who has FASD, can have problems in the domains of cognitive, behavioral, emotional, and social adaptation.

These are likely the youngsters who do not consistently focus their eye gaze on objects or persons. Individuals that seldom look others in the eye, do not pick up on all those expressive nuances necessary for understanding others, for developing empathy. Youngsters that can't think through the consequences of their behavior, established from observations of another person's behavior that allow them to understand that person's feelings: can't monitor their behavior based on empathy with others; based on realizing their behavior will impact others.

In kindergarten we expect children to develop social skills such as helping, cooperating, negotiating, and talking to solve interpersonal problems. At about age six, most children begin to acquire a conscience, internalizing moral rules of behavior and respect for individual differences. Self-monitoring is a beginning step in the development of self-control and social skills. The early preschool years are crucial to the acquisition of tools and strategies for social behavior.

CHALLENGING BEHAVIORS IN THE CLASSROOM

In 1985 when Beth Caruso, an experienced special education teacher, saw her first drug effected youngster she was "stunned by the student's lack of impulse control." Bouncing around the classroom with excess motor energy, he was unable to stay in his seat no matter what incentive to stay seated she used. Once his off-task behavior started, this youngster was unable to interrupt the behavior, unable to get back on track. Youngsters she has taught since bring these and other concerns.

A lack of social skills is compounded by behavioral unpredictability, "You can't predict what these youngsters will do next." Unlike the abused youngster with an explosive temper set off by a specific event, these youngsters can have outbursts without the heat of emotion, for no reason, or reasons apparently unconnected to recognizable events in the environment.

Youngsters who lack empathy with others are unable to see the other person's point of view. The most worrisome social behavior of youngsters with FASD/FDE may be the lack of judgment to respond to social rules; they could find themselves in a socially dangerous situation due to their lack of social judgment and indiscriminate trust. Many youngsters with FASD are easily influenced and "touchy," wanting to touch everyone, opening the door to inappropriate social behavior. Robin Lindsley has concerns that these children do not have self-protective responses. Unable to watch out for their own safety, they remain in jeopardy throughout life. Anyone can tell her student Jim to do something and he just does it.

It scares Beth Caruso that "these students give strangers hugs and follow strangers, they seem so open and need touch." This lack of social judgment paints a dangerous picture of youngsters growing into adulthood, liable to hurt others or be hurt by others. Mary Smith, an academic evaluation specialist, is concerned about their susceptibility to "con" men. Because of their lack of common sense about personal space, they may be sexual targets. All of the teachers I interviewed were concerned about the lack of social judgment their students would have as adults.

INSTRUCTIONAL STRATEGIES FOR LEARNING BEHAVIORS

The first step in a successful instructional program is matching your behavioral expectations with the level of the child's behavioral maturity level. Behaviors that require management and attention include: behavioral unpredictability, lack of empathy with others, lack of patience, hyperactivity, lack of inhibition, distracting others, and difficulty dealing with change. This variety of behaviors, including tantrums and violence, challenge classroom management.

Adults find it's easier to accept negative behaviors when they understand that the behaviors reflect an underlying pathology. Rather than focusing behavioral goals on functioning up to age level, focus in terms of management. Just as a diabetic has to manage medication and food, the person with FASD/FDE needs an environment that directs and supports, that provides appropriate activities and recreational experiences. Companionship based on friendship, nonprofessional companionship: just imagine how it would feel to have all your interpersonal contacts from the pool of professionals paid to help you.

The social comparisons, upon which one develops the perspectives needed for successful interpersonal interactions, may be too subtle. (Literally, teach specific behaviors and when to use them.) Support development of self-control in children by modeling correct behavior: redirecting, practicing, and setting clear limits. Behavior that the teacher models and rewards other students for is more likely to be imitated. Model the behaviors you expect the youngster to do.

Behavior rehearsal and role-play offer excellent methods to teach conflict resolution strategies and social behaviors. Role playing of appropriate behavioral options for a specific conflict situation include: walking away, talking, and negotiating. First, have the child use a successful strategy, then have other youngsters imitate that child's behavior. Conversation and group discussions that follow role-play activities, develop invaluable group support for specific adaptive social behaviors. Teach conflict resolution strategies on the playground, at the activity workstation, during free time, where the skills are used. Instruction in the specific situations where skills are used help compensate for a youngsters limited ability to generalize.

Explain the communication intent of others: what a look, body language, or gesture mean. Verbally labeling their own, the child's, and others' expressions of emotion, helps the child learn to identify those emotions. Interpreting social interactions may need to be taught in addition to social behaviors and appropriate emotional expressions.

> I never place a student in a yes/no situation, "I'll never win." (Meredith Anderson; kindergarten teacher)

Never get into win-lose situations. Provide several choices. Meredith Anderson, a kindergarten teacher never places her students in yes/no situations: "I'll never win." When making demands, she gives several choices. She recommends teachers "keep lessons short and transitions smooth." Teachers and parents find physical management a successful tool to keep youngster's behavior organized and under control: put your arms around them, take them by the hand, and recognize preschoolers may need to sit next to an adult. Meredith Anderson avoids problems by having the child sit next to her or a responsible child, during circle time activities that are not too stimulating. Some games are too exciting, and students become "wild." She finds time-out, working in a quiet area away from the whole group or stressful situation, provide the child with a procedure for respite when feeling overwhelmed. Olson (2002), using research from children of alcoholics, suggests interventions directed toward limiting stressors and increasing the protective factors of safety, stability, and predictability.

Play

Developmentally stimulating play nourishes imagination in physical, intellectual and social development; opening the door to all kinds of learning. Functional and symbolic aspects of cognitive development begin with children's play. Normal play moves from solitary, to standing by others watching, to cooperative play. Early play activities connect visual, tactile, and kinesthetic motor input. While engaging in manual tasks children visually attend, observing and learning from their play efforts. Curiosity and fun motivate further play exploration.

Youngsters with impaired play skills miss the intellectual and social benefits: the delight, derived from imaginative explorative early play learning experiences. The play of some children with FASD/FDE is not purposeful, not meaningful. They cannot organize their own play, cannot select materials, and may not be able to recognize or engage in the functional use of toys. Their play may consist of scattering, batting, picking up and putting down toys. Youngsters may *perseverate*, repeating the same action, for example, hitting a toy car against the wall over and over. They may become preoccupied with an object: staring at it, holding it, manipulating it. Children may show little interest in toys, with aimless wandering the play activity of choice.

Children may need to be taught how to play, may need to be taught the functional use of a few toys. For example, bring the toy to the child and wait for the child to recognize it. Respond immediately to any attempt to play or behave as if the child is responding, as if the child were beginning to play (Norris 1991). Educators can find out what is available in the child's home and include the same toys in classroom activities. Adult modeling of play and imitation of the child's play increases participation in play directed at exploring functional use of toys. Responding to and following the child's lead entices him/her to use their imagination. Modeling play and the functional use of toys for the child, using physical demonstration together with verbal descriptions begins development of the information processing strategies needed to integrate early social, intellectual, and physical learning experiences. Use of games like Simon Says that require imitation help youngsters follow directions and copy physical behaviors. A mom who adopted two siblings with FASD was shocked when I told her play activities may have to be taught just like other activities: hours had been spent taking toys out–then putting them back in the toy box.

Music was the only activity three-year-old Alan successfully participated in. Despite apparent similarities, the processes for the perception of music are different from those for spoken sounds (Luria 1970a). Skinny and misshapen, all head, elbows, and knees, Alan had frequent *petit mal* (brief, 10 second loss of most motor activity and awareness) seizures resulting in many falls. He was visually impaired, with few language or speech skills. Physical and intellectual disabilities compromised Alan's efforts at every turn. Yet, during music he would smile, come to his chair right away, sing, handle musical instruments, follow motor/music directions, and participate eagerly. As if he forgot to fuss, to get up and move away, to hit other kids! Music may be a pathway for participation, facilitating a range of skill practice and learning for some.

BRAIN MEDIATION OF BEHAVIOR

Focused and unfocused attention, monitoring the environment for significant events and possible dangers, even though not currently task relevant, is an essential part of adaptive behavior. Evidence suggests threat-related stimuli may be processed automatically, independent of attention, in the amygdala region of the brain (Dolan and Vuilleumier 2003).

Functional neuroimaging has found evidence suggesting a distinction between emotion and other forms of cognition, based on activation of the amygdala when subjects are shown faces with a fearful expression (Calder, Lawrence, and Young 2001). The youngster with damage to areas of the brain affecting attention or emotional information processing, as many youngsters with FASD do, just cannot recognize a dangerous situation. How often have we relied on these warnings just below consciousness, a sense "something is wrong," and adjusted our behavior. Moving one foot out of the way just in time to miss the falling box, or choosing a different street to walk down: ". . . emotional arousal organizes and coordinates brain activity" (LeDoux 2002). Fear responses can be triggered from fear-related stimuli that is difficult to understand and control. Even if we don't realize we are learning, our unconscious brain is working, is learning.

Billie McKenzie, R.N., a health coordinator for Portland Public Schools Head Start school nurses, has taken care of her 15-year-old grandson, Jamal, since birth. His mother took heroin, her addiction damaged Jamal in the womb, and controlled her life so that she was unable to parent. Billie describes Jamal as having "no memory." He has "autistic-like" flat affect. With his poor memory "every day is like the first day." Because nothing seems to matter to him and he forgets, discipline is nearly impossible. The social motivations most of us rely on are not available for him.

Judgment regarding personal safety has been a problem. Many times Jamal has ridden his bicycle to the local shopping mall, forgotten it and walked home. At the age of thirteen, large areas of the mall undergoing major construction changes were fenced off with "Danger" signs. Jamal wandered around the mall building site and climbed up on a part of Nordstrom's roof that was under construction. Very unsafe, one of the highest roofs in the mall, once upon it he couldn't get down. Jamal can't predict the consequences of his actions into the future. He didn't pay attention to the printed "Danger" warning signs, unable to generalize, maybe he couldn't recognize the word "Danger" when it wasn't printed on a large flash card presented to him by his teacher.

Police helped get Jamal down. Driving to the mall after the police called her to come pick up Jamal, Billie reevaluated her fears: can she ever safely leave him alone? Will he ever be able to handle unsupervised situations? She can't be there all the time.

> Consequences don't work with youngsters who forget the consequences.

Youngsters with FASD/FDE may not understand cause and effect. For example, putting your hand in a dog's eye makes the dog bite you: they forget about the dog bite and do it again. To reduce the incidence of unsafe behaviors, talk the child through the consequences of an action in brief concrete terms, and role-play cause and effect experiences: especially when there is uncertainty about which social rules to employ. Environments need to be protective, we can't expect the child to have a protective response.

Because of their poor choices and "seeming lack of fear," unable to project into the future what will happen when they do something, these youngsters can't be left alone. For example, a medical foster mom described a youngster who repeatedly put his hand on a hot stove, and didn't remember not to do it again. Because of unpredictable behavior, we can't anticipate what they will do. *Routines* can be followed to help children keep themselves healthy and safe. Children without self protective responses should not be expected to supervise themselves.

SUPPORT-THERAPY FOR CAREGIVERS

Counselors and therapists are needed to help parents find techniques and strategies: to manage their child, to deal with their own feelings, and to keep balance within the family. Biological mothers need to reduce their sense of guilt. Medical foster moms ask themselves, "Am I willing to live like that?" A mom finds she gets so tired she has trouble being charitable. How do parents deal with their anger and the anger of other children in the family? How can the family's strengths be rallied to adapt and cope?

Many behaviors are especially difficult to deal with, such as stealing, biting, and clinging. A medical foster mom advises, you have to remember "they didn't choose to be the way they are." Medical foster moms describe, they are never alone, youngsters have to be close to an adult constantly. Adults must literally, "watch out or you'll step on them." Youngsters don't recognize personal boundaries. One helps his mother drink her coffee. Particularly difficult is the lack of social judgment in combination with poor memory: "They forget you're mad."

Society's focus on therapy for the dysfunctional family has made many parents feel guilty unfairly, without addressing the practical needs of a family dealing with a chronic, twenty-four-hour-a-day, situation. Nancy grappled with the decision to remove her 13-year-old adopted son, John, from the family. His needs were becoming greater than the family's resources to meet those needs. The therapist working with Nancy told her "If you remove John, you will just find some other child to be the disruptive child." Youngsters with FASD/FDE can be in dysfunctional families, but neurological damage and the combination of defects these youngsters present, pose a set of daily living management problems for caregivers. Don't assume these youngsters can be introspective. Solution: a therapeutic focus on basic practical problem solving–change the behavior.

Deficits resulting from prenatal drug exposure are evident from the first day of life, before the environment has had an influence (Streissguth et al. 1989). When sensory input is biologically restricted, normal responses to stimuli break down. Emotion, human nature, is largely the product of the anatomic structure of ones' brain. Dr. Restak asks "What is the nature of the reality that our brains are capable of experiencing?" He explains "We behave the way we do because we are endowed with a brain which enables us to have certain experiences, think certain thoughts, and carry out certain actions that seem desirable" (Restak 1979). Behavior is determined by what is perceived, the neurological capacity to understand the information, and the range of responses available. Biologically determined mental limitations are not as easily taken into consideration as are physical limitations that we readily recognize. The impact of brain anatomy and function on behavior must be considered. Some deficits are so resistant to remedial efforts, the initial deficits youngsters experience may compound over the years, spilling over into all areas of their lives.

Chapter 4

INFANT

Practical techniques for fragile infant care are described in this chapter. For instance, how to filter out stimuli to help an infant focus, so that the sensory information required for development can be perceived and integrated. The easily overstimulated inconsolable infant is at risk for attachment-bonding problems. Similarities between descriptions of attachment-bonding disorders and descriptions of the behaviors of youngsters with FASD/FDE are pointed out.

ATTACHMENT AND BONDING

Foster Cline describes an arousal-relaxation attachment-bonding cycle, with gratification of the infant's needs by the parent. The stages of this cycle are: need, rage reaction (displeasure), gratification (satisfy need) or relief, and finally trust (Cline 1979). Parent-child interaction is initiated by the child's expression of displeasure and completed by the parent's response satisfying the child's need. As long as discomfort is present, the infant's attention is taken up with his/her immediate perceptions. When the outside world does not satisfy babies needs, without satisfying parent-child interactions, the infants ability to learn trust is jeopardized. As a result, the intellectual, physical and psychological development that is dependent upon these bonding perceptions is obstructed. Trust develops from having this cycle fulfilled.

Infants with FASD/FDE and others with health problems are at risk of having this cycle broken. They have pain the parent can't remove. Their difficult temperament may push the parent away, making it even more difficult for attachment to occur (Magid and McKelvey 1987). Unattached youngsters have not developed an understanding of cause and effect. When I'm hungry, I cry and someone feeds me. When I'm wet, I cry and someone changes me. If this early cause and effect learning is disrupted, the world looks chaotic.

The list of symptoms that describe unattached children contains many of the same behaviors found on lists describing the behaviors of youngsters with FASD/FDE.

Table 7. Signs and Symptoms of Lack of Attachment that Apply to Descriptions of Youngsters with FASD/FDE

- Lack the ability to give and receive affection
- Have trouble with basic cause and effect
- Have confused thought processes
- Lack long-term friends
- Have trouble recognizing their own feelings
- Have difficulty recognizing others feelings
- Have difficulty expressing feelings appropriately; especially anger, sadness, and frustration
- Self-destructive behavior
- Cruelty to others
- Phoniness
- Stealing, hoarding
- Preoccupation with fire, blood and gore
- Lack internal controls
- Abnormal eye contact
- Parents appear angry and hostile toward the child
- Superficial social skills and attractiveness
- May not show normal anxiety
- Lying
- May not show guilt
- May project blame on others
- Learning disorders
- Speech and language problems

Signs and symptoms of attachment disorder (Cline 1979; Fahlberg 1991; Magid and McKelvey 1987).

Parent-infant bonding interactions can be seriously compromised when a baby is demanding, irritable and unpredictable, yet unresponsive to comforting attempts. Visual and auditory avoidance in response to overstimulation, in addition, to deficits in the baby's ability to respond to the human face and voice contribute to poor bonding. These can be extremely difficult babies to parent, and less rewarding to caregivers; which put them at increased risk of being abused, of developing attachment disorders, or of being exposed to other drugs.

The drug/alcohol effected newborn's environment, with it's multiple caregivers: foster care, maternal psychopathology, and the chaos of the drug subculture, contribute to problems with bonding. Newborns prenatally drug/alcohol effected are born into physical and environmental circumstances that can jeopardize the attachment/ bonding process for them. Parenting from multiple caregivers contributes additional risks; when children receive uneven parenting, development of important attachments are jeopardized.

From infancy some youngsters with FDE dislike being touched. These noncuddlers lack social responses and smiles. They rarely laugh. They will not engage you with coy smiles, if they're overstimulated, you may be responded to with gaze aversion and a lack of facial expression. "Only a few of the drug-exposed toddlers displayed the interactive behaviors that are typically expected at this age, such as greeting and moving closer, and seeking close physical contact with the caregiver when she returns after a short separation. The majority of the drug-exposed children did not show the strong feelings of pleasure, anger, or distress. For the most part they remained affectively neutral" (Rodning, Beckwith, and Howard 1989). Their flat affect and avoidance behaviors hinder bonding and attachment.

Our tendency is to respond in kind. Someone smiles at us, we give them a smile in return. Someone says something nice; we say something nice in return. Joan Marguis, a social worker for early child intervention classrooms, is concerned about the adult who stops talking to the infant because the infant is not responding. Adults do things differently when they do not talk. For instance, how does an adult act when changing diapers without talking. Adults are likely to feel ineffective, to turn away from babies that do not become completely alert or babies that may change rapidly from one state to another, from sleep to crying. Babies who do not cry when they are hungry or wet, may not be fed or tended to appropriately (Brazelton and Cramer 1991). Commonly, adults adjust their response to the child's level, like mothers "baby-talk," the mutual imitation of adults and babies. Adults that care for these infants must ignore this instinct for a reciprocal response, must counteract their normal reaction to unresponsive infants that do not talk, demonstrate interest, laugh, or smile; and engage in a level of stimulation geared to the infant's/child's tolerance level. It was found that, offspring of mothers who provide high levels of support exhibit better coping skills and more secure attachment relations, based on maternal self-report of 42 biological mothers (O'Connor, Kogan, and Findlay 2002).

Imitate/model the signals, rhythms, smiles, frowns, movements, and vocalizations of the infant. Imitate/model intensity together with behavior. Behave as if the child knows how to communicate, as if the child's actions have intentional meaning (Norris 1991). Interpret the infants signals aloud, e.g., "you want more juice." When teaching Christopher, an eight-year-old child that did not talk, diagnosed autistic, imitating his behavior made him look at me, made him smile a bit. He still didn't talk, but he indicated interest. Although hesitant and a bit confused at having someone copy his behavior, I believe I saw a twinkle in his eye. Learning is pleasurable.

The development of moral judgment is jeopardized for youngsters unable to attach, unable to internalize their parent's values. The cycle of parent-child interaction is disrupted when reward for behavior that pleases, behavior that reflects the parent's values, is thwarted. A child's sense of "who I am" is interfered with. Poor judgment, and a lack of emotional development can result (Cline 1979; Fahlberg 1991; Magid and McKelvey 1987). To prevent the exacerbation of initial neurobehavioral impairments: when the newborn is discharged from the hospital the biological or foster parents need information about the newborn's diagnosis, specifics about what to expect and how to handle the infant.

Medical foster care is a resource for the hospitals that have abandoned fragile newborns requiring medical care, as overhospitalized babies demonstrate behaviors similar to the neglected child. The newborn's negative behaviors, screaming, withdrawing, regurgitating, can cause the nurses to withdraw: babies get less and less attention. Hospitals, particularly the Intensive Care Unit, contribute an emotionally negative environment. Stable families provide the optional combination in terms of safety and security for physical, intellectual, and psychological development.

Conventional wisdom I hear quoted in Children Services Division (CSD) circles is that once an infant has made an attachment, that youngster can be moved into another foster care placement, and be able to reattach. Many youngsters with FASD/FDE do not live with their biological parents. Of the nineteen children seen for assessment at the Clinical Training Unit's Diagnostic Clinic of the Child Development and Mental Retardation Center at the University of Washington and at the Holly Ridge Development Center, only four were living with their biological mothers. Fifteen were living with relatives or in foster care (Kieckhefer and Dinno 1992). When looking at ophthalmologic abnormalities Stromland and Hellstrom (1996) also looked at the social status of 25 children in Sweden with FASD, age range 4 to 19 years, median age 11 years. They found, the child living with: mother 4, with father or relative 6, in foster home 13, in institution 2; mother dead 10. Streissguth and colleagues (1991) evaluated 61 adolescents and adults who had been diagnosed FAS (70%) or had FAE (30%) in a patient follow-up study. "Most of the patients (77%) did not live with either biologic parent on follow-up: 26 percent were in foster homes, 21 percent with relatives, 16 percent adopted, and 9 percent in group homes or institutions. Only 5 percent lived alone but none were fully self-sufficient" (Streissguth et al. 1991).

Although multiple family placements can jeopardize attachment, in addition to intellectual and behavioral development, a stable non-biological home has been found to be beneficial. A study of 60 children prenatally exposed to alcohol found that mental and language development improved for children placed in foster care (Autti-Ramo et al. 1992). Rodning and colleagues (1989) studied the influence of attachment as reflected by secure and insecure feelings with a sample of 18 toddlers, 18 months old, prenatally exposed to a variety of drugs including cocaine, heroin, methadone, and phenylcyclidine hydrochloride (PCP); who lived in a variety of child rearing environments including foster care, extended family care, and with biological mothers. "The highest percentage of insecure drug-exposed toddlers was in the subgroup being raised by their biological mothers. In all cases but one, these mothers continued to abuse drugs. The majority of drug-exposed toddlers reared by extended family members and foster mothers were secure" (Rodning et al. 1989).

Table 8. Attachment Helps the Child to . . .

- Attain intellectual potential
- Attain psychological potential
- Develop social skills
- Trust others
- Cope with stress and frustration

Parent-infant relationships in the first years of life influence both physical and intellectual development together with forming the foundation for psychological development.

MATERNAL CRIMINAL RESPONSIBILITY

Infants prenatally exposed to cocaine usually do not die. Yet, these medically, neurologically, and nutritionally compromised newborns may not be able to function even with medical attention and care. Ms. Green's baby died two days after birth because of her use of cocaine. The county coroner, P. John Seward MD, described the cause of death this way: ". . . cocaine ingested by Green traveled through the placenta to her fetus, reducing the oxygen supply and causing brain damage. Further injury was caused when the placenta prematurely ruptured, leaving the baby without sufficient blood and oxygen. The baby's brain swelled, and her heart eventually stopped while in Rockford Memorial Hospital's pediatric high-risk unit . . ." (Somerville 1989). In 1989 the courts, dealing with the case brought against Ms. Green, grappled with the issue of whether a mother can be held criminally responsible for her actions that damage the fetus. The Illinois grand jury refused to indict Ms. Green, the first woman, charged with involuntary manslaughter (ibid). The future may find that fetal rights take precedence over maternal rights.

Maternal vulnerability differences, range from economic and educational; to the individual genetics of alcohol metabolic efficiency, which cause differences in maternal drinking behavior and in fetal vulnerability. How can the courts punish women when society has not first offered treatment? Although the Supreme Court has recognized addiction is an illness, will mothers come in for prenatal care if they're afraid they'll be put in jail? How much does the average child-bearing aged woman know about the law?

Keep in mind that when in a threatening situation we automatically limit the range and amount of information we have to deal with. Spend a few seconds in an addicted persons shoes: imagine how you would feel if you were walking down the street with cocaine in your pocket. Are you hypervigilant—are you afraid? In the *Ferguson v City of Charleston* (2001) case, the Supreme Court found that pregnant women could not be subjected to drug testing for the purpose of criminal prosecution, without a warrant or explicit consent.

FRAGILE INFANT CARE

Medical foster mothers care for newborns that are not strong enough to survive. Infants with respiratory abnormalities and altered brainstem responses that regulate arousal, may be at risk for Sudden Infant Death Syndrome (SIDS). Newborns that die from SIDS or from *apnea*, failure to breath, die in their sleep without monitors to alert parents when breathing stops. These fragile newborns who have sleep related deficits in arousal may need to be on a monitor. Compounding their physical hurdles; some infants are hypersensitive to sound, and the monitor can damage the hairs in their ears. Ruth Stroemple, an infant care specialist who trains medical foster care mothers, recommends reducing stimulation: cover the crib with a blanket, dim the lighting, quiet the environment for sound, use music with a heartbeat in the background to help the infant sleep comfortably. Replacing good infant care with vigilant extraordinary care can minimize the expression of teratologic effects.

The fragile infant doesn't, or can't generate the responses to get what it needs. For example, the baby can't suck, can't console itself, can't self-protect. In addition, internal organization and control is compromised by the newborn's physical limitations. This infant may require more stimulation to become aroused and attentive, but then may quickly become overaroused. Ruth Stroemple recommends, attention needs to be paid to developing internal organization in an environment that is consistent and predictable. Introduce and practice new activities when the baby is calm. Be predictable. Use the same procedures consistently, the baby does not tolerate a variety of methods. Once a smooth routine is established, do everything the same way each time. Use a fixed routine for feeding, bathing, and sleeping. Babies needs time to anticipate and organize themselves. Tell the baby what you're doing "I'm moving you," then move slowly. Give the baby as much freedom as you can within safe, predictable limits. Interpret babies signals aloud, e.g., "you want some more." Introduce information, sounds, textures, and sights slowly and cautiously throughout the day. When sufficient time to respond is available and the activity is readily predictable, success is increased. A normal baby can hear and see best at about eight to ten inches away from the babies chest. Present visual information at the correct range: if eight inches is the infants visual range, don't show things at ten inches. Bring objects to the baby's midline. Babies do not reach for toys that are not close enough. Babies like faces and high contrast bright shiny toys. Eye contact is more easily achieved if adults keep their face within the babies direct line of vision. Watching an object requires of the baby sufficient motor skill and coordination to move the head, together with the suppression of irrelevant motor responses. Infants with FASD/FDE are likely to have difficulty organizing and controlling movement.

Failure-to-thrive newborns look gaunt, with a large head, sparse hair, and dry skin. They have no fat pads on their bottom, just saggy skin. Tactile hypersensitivity to the feeling of milk in their mouth and a poor appetite present unusual feeding challenges. The first six months are crucial for catch-up growth. Failure-to-thrive babies should gain two pounds per month, Ruth Stroemple recommends holding to get infants over the practice of regurgitation; hold them for twenty minutes after feeding. Babies may need to be swaddled and comforted with slow vertical rocking. Poor feeding is dangerous; fragile infants need extra calories. For instance, the infant who has difficulty feeding may have disabilities like cerebral palsy that produce a requirement for extra calories. Infants may be intolerant to milk. In the intestine, the enzyme that is the first to be lost after diarrhea and is the last to be replaced is the enzyme needed to digest lactose. Change from milk formula to a soy-based formula, while the enzyme is building up again. Feeding tip: for babies that can't suck, that can't close their mouth over a nipple; put your finger under the infants chin while rubbing it's cheeks to stimulate sucking. For babies that never seem to mouth things, try putting a dab of baby food on a toy. Good health and development require compensation techniques to overcome the ramifications of feeding difficulties.

Sensory Stimulation

The human brain growth spurt spans the last trimester of pregnancy to several years after birth. At birth the brain is about one fourth the size of an adult brain. Brain cell neurons grow in size, the number of axons, dendrites, and synaptic sites increase. The maturing nervous system needs stimulation to modify and fine-tune itself, for neurons to develop specificity (Shatz 1992). This development is dependent on sensory and motor stimulation. The challenge is to get the hypersensitive infant to accept stimulation.

IQ increases with stimulation. In the brain the cerebral cortex is the most changed with either a stimulating or an impoverished environment (Rosenzweig, Bennett, and Diamond 1972). Studies of rats give clues to the impact enriched or impoverished environments can have on human beings. Enriched environments produced greater weight and thickness in the rats' cerebral cortex. In addition, enriched environments produced larger cell bodies, and nuclei with synapses much larger than those in their littermates who were given an impoverished environment (Rosenzweig et al. 1972). Early deprivation, may have effects similar to those of brain injury deficits (Reynolds 1981). Infant stimulation provides sensory enrichment to fully develop the senses that are intact, to develop early perceptual patterns.

The hippocampus, critical in memory formation, is "turned on" by novelty (Restak 1979). Recordings made of single cells in the hippocampus of rats show that they fire selectively in response to changes in the environment: slower discharges when animals are immobile, and rapid cell discharges when animals are exploring new environments. The brain structures thought to be most involved in memory formation are the cerebellum, hippocampus, amygdala, and cerebral cortex (Thompson 1986; Restak 1979).

Can the infant with FASD/FDE benefit from enriched stimulation? The internal and external feedback system necessary for perceptual development and organization is compromised in infants who have a low threshold for stimulation; hence are unresponsive to stimuli. The infant with a limited ability to inhibit irrelevant input, easily overwhelmed by sensory stimulation, needs information presented *within—at the threshold of,* that infant's unique sensory parameters. For example, a small spice jar filled with rice may make a more tolerable rattle sound than the harsher sounds of a babies rattle. These infants need help to focus attention, so they can learn perceptual and organizational skills other infants acquire automatically.

The literature on infant stimulation support medical foster moms who stress the importance of a calm atmosphere as a starting point. The amount of stimulation/information must be kept to a tolerable amount. Babies may calm best to only one form of stimulation at a time, and instead of rocking and singing, try only rocking. "Time-out" periods at the first signs of stress help infants regain enough organization to focus on and respond to stimuli.

Techniques to reduce stimulation include tightly swaddling the infants, holding their hands to midline, giving them pacifiers, placing them in foam contour chairs, and rocking them gently in a rounded vertical position. Posture is critical for infants with excessive muscle tone. For example, holding the baby in a rounded tilted forward position helps stop stiff rounded backward arching and other abnormal posturing. If eye contact is overstimulating for the baby to tolerate, have the baby face away from you. Many of these infants need considerable assistance to maintain self-control when they receive stimulation (Chasnoff 1989). Nonintrusive stimuli can be used to develop the control of attention and suppression of interfering reflexes that is needed to accept stimuli essential for development.

"Babies won't imitate complex actions they don't understand themselves" (Gopnik, Meltzoff, and Kuhl 1999). Normal babies have basic knowledge principles to help understand the world, for example, how objects move. Young babies can follow the movements of an object in front of them and be able to predict how an object will move in the future. A ball rolling on a table rolls behind a screen, and the baby will look ahead to the far edge, where the ball ought to appear (Gopnik et al. 1999).

Sound imitation is when the baby makes a sound with a toy or object, then you imitate the sound baby made with a similar object. If baby changes actions, imitate the changes. Show how objects can made different sounds if they are banged against different surfaces. Vary the sound a little, e.g., if you've been imitating baby banging a block on the highchair tray, after a few times, bang the block on a can.

Never Shake Baby

When shaken, a baby's soft brain bumps back and forth against the skull. Permanent brain damage can be caused from bruising and intracranial hemorrhage. The combination of a heavy head, weak neck muscles, a soft brain, a thin skull, together with the lack of head and neck mobility and control make newborns extremely vulnerable to injury from shaking. The brain stem, frontal lobe, and temporal lobes are particularly vulnerable. Doctor John Caffey first described the shaken baby syndrome, in 1972. Shaken babies are often under six months of age (Spaide 1990). The inconsolable crying of the cocaine/polydrug effected newborn puts them in jeopardy of provoking this behavior in parents/caregivers who are unaware of the possible damage. Wire the babies brain with emotionally positive sensory learning experiences such as touch, taste, sight, sound, smell. Babies develop an extra sense "Baby knows how you feel about him" (Ruth Stroemple, infant care specialist).

STIMULATING HOME ENVIRONMENTS

The quality of the caregiving environment has the strongest influence on infants development. Frank and colleagues (2002) found infants prenatally cocaine-exposed with a low birth weight that are placed with kinship caregivers are at increased risk for less optimal development outcomes. Brown, Bakeman, Coles, Platzman and Lynch (2004) also found 41 percent out of 83 cocaine-using mothers in their study, relinquished care of their children. Children placed in nonrelative foster or adoptive care lived in homes with more stimulating environments and had caregivers with better vocabulary scores (Singer, et al. 2004). Arendt and colleagues (2004) are in agreement with Singer "The most useful predictors of outcome measures in all regressions proved to be maternal vocabulary score (PPVT-Revised) and home environment at age 7 years." Maternal/caregiver reading level has been found to be predictive of school readiness for prenatally drug-exposed youngsters (Pulsifer, Radonovich, Belcher, and Butz 2004). Enriched environments were reflected in the higher verbal IQs of adoptive and foster mothers, than for maternal and biologic caregivers (Lewis, et al 2004). The recommendation suggested here is to design interventions that improve both the mother's caregiving and academic skills.

Consistent with this kinship data is my personal experience on the Citizens Review Board with relatives caring for infants known to have prenatal drug exposure. The predominant comment was that the infants were doing their best, especially considering the negative environment they came from. All kinship caregivers were optimistic, given that most if not all of these infants were "beautiful babies" with no visible deformities, environment was seen as the only problem of concern—not biology. These kinship caregivers were not customarily given the infant stimulation training the medical foster moms were.

Schuler, Nair, and Kettinger (2003) found that a home intervention with drug-exposed infants and their biological mothers through 18 months of age, was superior for infants whose mothers discontinued drug use after their infant's birth. Part of this home intervention protocol, weekly for the first six months then biweekly (lasting about 28 minutes); was having home visitors explain age-appropriate developmental skills using games and activities, focusing on the parent then the infant. Some parents have learning disabilities themselves and need information presented with the same instructional strategies as their children. Also, parents have described becoming so emotionally overwhelmed when dealing with professionals regarding their child, that focusing on relevant information was overtaken with confusion. Teach parents strategies one idea at a time, present information slowly with repetition. Accepting affectionate home environments with a variety of language stimulation experiences as well as physical experiences geared to the youngsters developmental level, provide the supportive foundation for productive community and school experiences.

PART II

Chapter 5

COGNITIVE PROCESSES

Basic neurological concepts involved in learning are described in this chapter: neurobiology, neuroplasticity, and hemisphere specialization. Normal cognitive processes provide us with a comparative basis to understand the impact of damage. Scientific knowledge, unheard of a few decades ago, increases in understanding neuroanatomy, the neural organization and neurobiological functions of the brain, contribute to targeting therapeutic options that focus on reducing the effects of prenatal toxic drug/alcohol exposure.

NEUROIMAGING WINDOWS

Neuroimaging techniques allow study of the structure and the functioning of active brains. Positron emission tomography (PET), magnetic source imaging (MSI), and functional magnetic resonance imaging (fMRI) utilize the fact that active neurons have a higher metabolism. The noninvasive fMRI measures blood flow and oxygenation. Voxel-based morphometry (VBM) imaging looks at the whole brain in three dimension. The noninvasive MSI allows for visualization of activated brain regions based on the localization of electrical currents in neurons. The PET scans for areas of the brain that are burning glucose, after radioactive glucose is injected.

No longer do neurologists have to study brains from autopsy. Structural neuroimaging along with functional imaging techniques have proven to be invaluable for understanding which brain regions are effected in FASD, and how functioning is effected (Riley, Guerri, et al. 2003). Not all researchers are as optimistic, Bhatara and colleagues (2002) found "Functional neuroimaging studies in FAS are difficult to undertake . . . the patients are so restless that they are unable to cooperate without sedation."

In addition to neuroimaging techniques, newer microscopic techniques, only a few years old, permit a greater resolution of tissue samples: ". . . the biology of memory can now be studied at two different levels, one aimed at nerve cells and the molecules within nerve cells, and the other aimed at brain structures, circuitry, and behavior" (Squire and Kandel 1999).

THE CHEMISTRY AND BIOLOGY OF MEMORY

There are an estimated one hundred billion neurons in the brain, each one predisposed to learning. The brain is designed to discover—to learn. "Like trails through the woods, neural networks become better established the more they are traveled" (Maranto 1984). Each neuron can store thousands of memories.

The major parts of the neuron are: the dendrite, the cell body, the axon, and the axons presynaptic terminals. The dendrite receives information, the cell body integrates information, and the axon transmits information. Each neuron can communicate with 100,000 or more other neurons by way of the synapse. Picture 100 billion neurons, a thicket, not really touching each other, connecting to transmit information at synaptic sites using neurotransmitters. There may be 50 different neurotransmitters. A typical synapse has three components: a presynaptic terminal, a postsynaptic target cell, and a small space in between these two processes, separating the two neurons. The axon impulse can travel distances from 0.1 millimeter to a meter or more, depending on the specific cell. In this biological impulse, an electrical current runs down the axon to the synaptic site: then a chemical neurotransmitter transmits information from one neuron to another across the synaptic gap. Neurons use two types of signals: a large all-or-none electrochemical called *action potential* for signaling within the neuron. The second type of signal called the *synaptic potential,* has the purpose of passing information from one neuron to another, at the synapse.

When Marian C. Diamond, examined sections of Albert Einstein's brain, she discovered a surprisingly large number of nonneuronal cells, known as glia, around neurons in the association cortex. This area, not surprisingly, is involved in high-level cognition. By the mid-1990s neuroscientists established that glia had a variety of receptors on their membranes that could respond to a range of chemicals, including, in some cases, neurotransmitters, and that glia influence the formation of synapses. Glial cells outnumber neurons nine to one. Previously, glia were thought to only nurture neurons. In the past several years, sensitive imaging tests have shown that neurons and glia engage in a two-way dialogue from embryonic development through old age (Fields, R.D. 2004).

Experience shapes our brain, cellular changes underlying learning involve modifying the physical and chemical properties of the neuron, an ongoing processes of reorganizing neural anatomy. The variety of neuronal transformations that can occur as a result of learning include structural and chemical alterations in synaptic transmission, greater dendritic branching, more spines, higher spine densities, and formation of new synapses. With learning, synapses change their shape and structure, chemical changes take place in protein synthesis and neurotransmitter receptors, also the amount of neurotransmitter released at the presynaptic terminal. In addition, synapses are lost through the "pruning" of unused neural connections. There is a short period (hours or days) in which cellular changes are reversible. Forgetting is part of learning new information, part of adapting to changes in information. These changes can permanently alter the neuron's response to a neurotransmitter. These biochemical processes interact with the environment, establishing, retaining, and triggering memories. Learning is dynamic, continually being modified by experience and practice: connections expand and retract as a result of how neuronal pathways are used over time. Individuals vary in the efficiency of brain cell communication.

Synaptic connections are excitatory or inhibitory: exciting the sites that receive information, and inhibiting sites that interfere. When filtering out irrelevant information, the electrochemical exchange of neural communication is more inhibitory than excitatory (Sylwester 1986). Neurons establish appropriate synaptic connections: each nerve cell innervates particular presynaptic cells, avoiding other potential synaptic partners that are incorrect. Cells are selective about what they respond to. The easily overstimulated child prenatally exposed to drugs/alcohol may have deficits in aspects of neural inhibition that make focusing attention especially difficult.

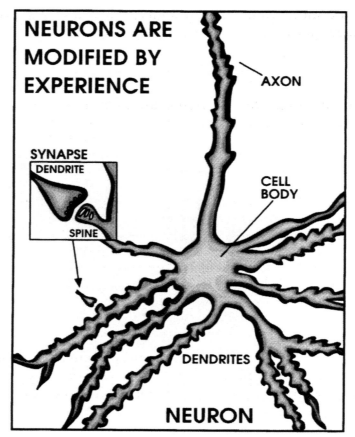

Figure 7. Neurons are modified by experience. (Designed by Paul Parker. With permission.)

NEUROPLASTICITY

Neuronal signals prevented from taking their appropriate route find another neuropathway. The name for this neuronal rerouting, mother natures recovery of function is called plasticity; *neuroplasticity*, the brains capacity to reorganize itself. This plasticity serves all of us: elderly stroke patients, accident victims, and newborns. The effect of damage is delayed if the damaged structure is not functionally mature and not utilized; also if the memory involves many brain regions, other nondamaged regions compensate. Actions can be carried out through a variety of pathways, substitutions of one area for another, one sense for another. The immature nervous system is generally considered to be more vulnerable to injury, but is also able to recover from damage that would be devastating to adults. An insult sustained at any particular point in the developmental ontological process has the potential to disrupt neural processes throughout the nervous system (Spear 1984).

Studies have suggested damage caused by prenatal alcohol exposure, may jeopardize plasticity, resulting in less recovery of function than seen in injury after birth (Connor, et al. 2000). The neurotransmitters that spark the series of molecular events necessary for memory retrieval may be disrupted. What is the content of a memory resulting from connections between damaged brain areas? What if memory for where and when is developed in a healthy area, and memory for facts is developed in a damaged area? Unfortunately, the recovery of function provided by neuroplasticity is not as available to youngsters that have central nervous system (CNS) damage. ". . . drugs provide a marked contrast, in producing notable and permanent disruption of CNS function" (Kuhn, Bero, Ignar, Lurie, and Field 1987). A large percentage of cells that produce norepinephrine (a neurotransmitter effected by cocaine) are located in the locus caeruleus, a primary center in the brain involved in plasticity. Thus, despite the compensatory processes during development, it is likely that recovery of function would not be complete for offspring prenatally exposed to drugs/alcohol.

What if one of the areas in the brain is damaged? The coordinated connections between neural systems break down, and participation in the damaged area is jeopardized. Thus, damage in one area can affect the functions of other systems and regions (LeDoux 2002). Atypical cognitive strategies may be found to compensate. Neuronal pathways can be changed; other structures in the brain, other neurons than were originally intended take over the functioning of damaged areas. Different strategies can be used to achieve a goal. The amount of cortical tissue damage effects both performance, and the degree of recovery possible.

Neuroplasticity involves a variety of growth, regeneration, and reinnervation avenues for damaged neurons. In addition, certain aspects of behavior survive brain damage. A new or different behavioral *strategy* can be used to compensate for a lost behavior. Nerve cells can become *supersensitive* resulting in increased responsiveness. *Regeneration*, regrowth of damaged neurons occurs. Dendrites increase branches to facilitate *reorganization*, establishing new connections for damaged neurons. *Rerouting*, neurons seek out new targets, new neurons to communicate with when their normal targets have been removed. *Supplemental* axons grow to replace lost axons or to innervate different neurons. Multiple neurological systems participate in a given behavior; thus, while one system may be damaged, the behavior can be continued with an alternate system.

Given that injury occurred before age two, neuroplasticity may have rerouted the pathways so no loss of skill would be recognized. Our brain reaches adult size by age twenty-one. Recovery potential is greater for a developing human nervous system than for a mature one, particularly sensory input and speech. Recovery of function from injury after age two will not be as extensive as if injury occurred before age two. The extent of impairment is dependent upon the overall health and the maturity of brain structures at the time of injury. Also, limited demands for a skill may delay the appearance of a deficit, in spite of damage. For instance, we don't expect a newborn to walk or talk, read or write, the child appears normal until more complex activities are expected. The prefrontal area, responsible for the performance of most intellectual tasks, is not psychologically active until a child is between five and eight-years-old. As a result, the effect of deficits resulting from early damage may not be seen until after eight years of age (Reynolds 1981). Each child presents a unique picture of damage reflecting the extent of insult to their brain. Looking at neuronal transmission: does the pathway work at all, does a different pathway work to relay the information, does only a part of the pathway work?

Development of the central nervous system involves stages of organization and function. First, neurons are born and migrate to their particular positions. Second, axons and dendrites develop patterns specific for different cell types. Then, specific synaptic connections between neurons are formed. Brain development continues after birth with different areas maturing at different times, complete maturation occurs around puberty.

Although the immature nervous system is more vulnerable to insult, it is protected with a greater potential to recover from damage, than does an adult's. Yet, the fetus exposed to drugs/alcohol may be at risk for disruption of the process of neuroplasticity, because the youngster may have permanent central nervous system deficits. In general, the more functionally intact neurological systems are, the more the effects of damage can be minimized (Golden 1981).

Recovery of function is uncertain, it may be immediate or delayed, transient or permanent. Neuronal rearrangement may be adaptive or maladaptive; structures are called upon to take over functions for which they were not originally intended. The brain works as an integrated system: when an area of the brain is destroyed, the person's behavior is being caused not by the damaged area, but rather by other structures in the brain that are performing in the absence of the damaged area.

LEFT AND RIGHT HEMISPHERES

Information is transferred between the left and right hemispheres, in the brain, by corpus callosum fibers that connect the hemispheres. Hemispheres are specialized to work with different types of information using different processing and different cognitive styles. The left hemisphere utilizes an analytical logical mode, suitable for words; the right utilizes a holistic style, suitable for spatial forms. Hemisphere disconnection, failures in processing might result from disturbances in the relations between the hemispheres (Gregory 1989; Restak 1979). Behavior disconnections may be based on disturbances of hemispheric specialization.

A vivid example of hemisphere differences was found in the classic study, conducted by Sperry, of split brain patients who had a severed corpus callosum. Words such as KEYCASE, were flashed onto a projection screen for one-tenth of a second or less, intervals too brief for the subjects to move their eyes. The letters KEY appeared only in the split-brain patient's left visual field, CASE appeared only in the right visual field. When the patients were asked what they had seen, they said they saw the word CASE, verbal skills are in the left hemisphere. The patients then inserted their left hand into a bag and, by touch alone, retrieved the object they had just seen flashed on the screen. They removed a KEY, motor skills are in the right hemisphere, even though the subjects said they had seen the word CASE (Restak 1979). Each hemisphere seems to have its own separate sensations, its own perceptions, and its own concepts.

Communication between hemispheres is established across fibers

Table 9. Left and Right Hemisphere Functions.

	Left Hemisphere		Right Hemisphere
Language:	articulating speech and comprehension of language		Recognition of emotions
			Nonverbal awareness
Math:	mathematical theory, computation		Music
Temporal:	sequencing one thing after another	Analogic:	recognizing likenesses, understanding metaphors
Rational:	drawing conclusions based on facts	Motor:	spatial skills, movement, motor learning, drawing
Logical:	drawing conclusions based on consistent reasoning	Intuitive:	making leaps of insight, often based on incomplete patterns, hunches, feelings, or visual cues
		Holistic:	perceiving whole overall patterns

(Kane 1984; Edwards 1979; Gregory 1989). Photo design: Kathy Bassett

of the corpus callosum connecting the left and right hemispheres. For example, emotional information from the right hemisphere is combined with the language information in the left hemisphere, by way of the corpus callosum. The corpus callosum is frequently smaller or almost nonexistent in youngsters with FASD. Neuroimaging with single photon emission computed tomography (SPECT), found reduced cerebral blood flow, which reflects neuronal activity, in three patients with FAS, suggesting impaired left hemisphere function (Bhatara et al. 2002). Using a task that required identification of which finger tips were touched, Roebuch, Mattson, and Riley (2002) found children with FASD had deficits in processing between the two cerebral hemispheres. In addition to corpus callosum functioning affecting learning and behavior, they found deficits became more pronounced as the tasks increased in complexity requiring a greater integration across the two cerebral hemispheres.

EXECUTIVE FUNCTIONS

Executive functioning describes the overarching organization and integration of cognitive processes involved with the problem-solving of tasks that do not involve familiar, well-learned information. These processes influence the quality of the completed task and if a task is completed at all. Executive functions incorporate the ability to utilize information contained in working memory and the *integration* of basic cognitive processes: motor, sensation, perception, attention, memory, and thus, depend on healthy cognitive development (Eslinger 1996).

Executive function can be defined as a group of higher level cognitive abilities that include (a) planning, the imitation and organization of goal-directed problem-solving behaviors (b) flexibility, the ability to adapt to unexpected circumstances, to change strategies, (c) hypothesis generation, (d) abstract reasoning, (e) control of attention despite distraction, (f) response inhibition, (g) sequencing of behaviors, (h) executing tasks simultaneously, (i) to place episodes in time and place, (j) self-regulation of behavior, (k) interpretation of emotions, and (l) obeying the rules of interpersonal social behavior. These abilities are used when retrieving relevant information from long-term memory and integrating it with new information in working memory.

Aspects of executive function are distributed throughout several cortical regions and spread across multiple regions of the frontal cortex (Carpenter, Just, and Reichle 2000). The prefrontal cortex, compromising about 30 percent of the entire cortex, keeps track of the time and the place information was acquired; simultaneously analyzes and integrates sensory information, providing the basis for the formation of intentions, the organization and implementation of actions. The prefrontal cortex receives connections from sensory systems, like the visual and auditory, enabling it to be aware of what's going on; from the hippocampus and other areas involved in long-term memory (LeDoux 2002). The outer layer of the brain, the prefrontal cortex, has six layers: the middle layers flavor receiving inputs while the deep layers send outputs. Youngsters that have prefrontal lobe damage exhibit deficiencies in their ability to use knowledge to guide their behavior in everyday situations (Goldman-Rakic 1992). ". . . Luria, pointed out two characteristic deficits of patients with damage to the frontal lobes: they lack spontaneous, purposeful behavior and they lack an understanding of their deficits" (LeDoux 2002). In summary, discrete prefrontal regions implement high-level cognitive processes that can serve to enhance memory encoding and subsequent long-term memory. Connor and colleagues (2000) note that although patients with FASD often have demonstrated problems with executive functioning: studies have not identified structural damage to the frontal lobe. Yet, it is predictable that structural or functional changes to the frontal lobes or to pathways that link frontal lobe functions with the rest of the brain will be found.

Short Term - Working Memory

Based on your own cognitive executive function adequacy; speculate, imagine, your own working memory is a box with connections to many other boxes. The box can hold ten items of a certain degree of difficulty. Information is looked at, manipulated, compared, and held easily when the box contains ten or less items. The temporary storage of information while processing incoming data is efficient. When the learning situation demands an eleventh item—the workload processing demands exceed the capability of the box.

Working memory integrates information about the present with memories from past experiences, and includes the current and past emotional content of those experiences, while keeping an overall goal in mind. Information placed in working memory, for example, can influence retrieval of information relevant to the demands of current circumstances: what we attend to, the way we see things, and the way we act.

Chapter 6

LEARNING

The study of cognition draws from a broad spectrum of disciplines: biology, philosophy, sociology, anthropology, linguistics, cognitive psychology, and neurosciences, to bring perspectives on learning and memory. Basic normal cognitive functional interactions among brain systems, as well as the cellular plasticity that underlie learning and memory, are presented in this chapter so that instructional options, for normal and atypical cognitive process, can be evaluated. Understanding the processes of learning influence the instructional decisions we make: choices supported by scientifically-based research, informed by neurology.

Youngsters damaged by prenatal drug/alcohol exposure are likely to have ineffective mental processes that disrupt the ability to extract and use information; whereas other youngsters automatically use effective information processing strategies, to organize and remember information. Although deficits may manifest globally and specifically, performance across domains is unlikely flat, with aspects of memory function relatively preserved. Performance is related to the type of task and the type of response required. Multiple memory processes support the physical and social interactions necessary for so many of our commonplace everyday functions. ". . . there are many forms of memory, that different brain structures carry out specific jobs, and that memory is encoded in individual nerve cells and depends on changes in the strength of their interconnections" (Squire and Kandel 1999).

The process of normal skill development from infancy through childhood reflects a pattern of sporadic skill acquisition: learning–loss of a skill–followed by reacquisition. A skill or concept must be relearned many times before acquisition is accomplished (Bower 1976). Youngsters with FASD/FDE have deficits that exacerbate this pattern of sporadic skill acquisition. Inconsistent use of problem-solving strategies, episodes of disorganization, and susceptibility to the effects of interference negatively complicate learning.

The process of learning is influenced by previous learning, cognitive ability, the ability to focus attention, and the information processing strategies of the learner. Using strategies to construct meaning, the brain actively perceives, selects, attends to, organizes, stores, and retrieves information (Heilman 1978). Learning causes physical modifications in brain structure and the brain's activity, so that we can perform some tasks automatically without thinking, without analysis (Luria 1970b). The capacity for learning is a function of the reciprocal relationship between the brain and behavior, ". . . the number of times the event or fact is repeated, its importance, the extent to which we can organize it and relate it to knowledge that we already have, and the extent to which we rehearse the material after it has first been presented" (Squire and Kandel 1999).

The brain organizes information it receives making mental constructions, comparing and adding new knowledge to existing information. New concepts are formed. Existing knowledge combines with new information creating concepts which extend the scope of information. Associations are established between information which already has meaning; linking it with kinesthetic, visual, auditory, and other sensations relevant to the current task. Existing knowledge plays a crucial role in remembering, selecting what is attended to, and interpreting information.

FORMATION OF MEMORY

Many memories can be produced from the same experience. What happens when we are presented with information? Sensory messages are perceived, interpreted, and responded to: (1) we search for the important elements of information, inhibiting irrelevant stimuli (2) we separate what is useful from what is unimportant (3) we compare new information with the information we already have in our long-term memory. With this we create a hypothesis regarding the whole (think about what your doing with this information) (4) we select a plan of response and decide if this new information will go into long-term memory. If we decide to place the new information into long-term memory, physical changes, memory-traces are generated in the neuron. Existing knowledge is always changing in response to the active process of examination and reformulation. Neurons are constantly updated and modified by new experiences resulting in large pathways of interconnected neurons: longer and branchier dendrites, changes in the size and strength of synapses.

Table 10.
Cognitive Processes: What Happens When We Are Presented with Information?

Sensory Messages are Perceived, Interpreted, and Responded to
I. PERCEIVE
A. Search for important elements of information
B. Inhibit responses to irrelevant stimuli
II. INTERPRET
A. Compare new information with established memories
B. Create a hypothesis
C. Verify this hypothesis by comparing it with new information
III. RESPOND
A. Storage: determine if new information is to be kept in long-term memory
B. Action: determine if new information prompts action now

(Luria 1970b; Heilman 1978)

The word *trace* refers to the physical basis of memory, the structural change in the neuron and glial cells resulting from learning. Thus, we can think of a trace as a bit of memory, a memory-trace, an engram. "The principle is that a declarative memory engram is distributed among different brain regions, and these regions are specialized for particular kinds of perception and information processing" (Squire and Kandel 1999). Memory appears to be stored in the same brain structures that originally perceived and processed the experience.

Conscious and Unconscious Memory

Many forms of memory can function in parallel. *Declarative* memory is a conscious memory, a memory for facts, ideas, and events. The operations of declarative memory include: encoding (how information is attended to, processed, and prepared for storage), storage, retrieval, and forgetting. *Nondeclarative* memory, an unconscious memory resulting from experience, involves the reflexive performance of various motor and perceptual skills, habituation, sensitization, and habits. Distributed across many brain systems these nondeclarative memories are unavailable to conscious awareness, but can affect functioning, evidenced in how we do something, for example, riding a bicycle. Thus, despite brain damage, there can be remarkably preserved functioning outside a person's awareness, in unconscious routes over which information is processed in the brain.

It is unlikely people consciously recall or recognize information and experiences they have not consciously attended to. Nevertheless, incidental nondeclarative learning occurs from unattended awareness. Incidental learning contributes to our fund of knowledge and may play an important part in our social learning, when information contains aspects that are not explicit in the material but inferred. For example, the listener moves back a step, the speaker recognizes the listener is uncomfortable and can adjust what they're saying, the subject, word choice, volume, and tone. Incidental learning, together with separating relevant from irrelevant information, is adversely effected by difficulties related to focusing attention (Eich 1984).

Memory Consolidation

To *consolidate*, the combining of information into a single unifying concept involves time and effort. First, it takes *time* to consolidate a memory-trace. Consolidation, the formation of a long-term memory takes place in synapses and individual neurons, developing only if new protein is synthesized; a coordinated structural change is required in both presynaptic and postsynaptic cells (Squire and Kandel 1999). Interference can disrupt this consolidation. For instance, accident victims who are unable to remember an accident may not have formed the memory-trace, there is just no conscious, declarative memory, no trace. If you're driving down street A and have an accident on street B, the accident interferes with consolidation of the memory-trace for what happened between street A and street B. Second, the learner must have a sufficient processing *effort* and focus of *attention* for a sufficient period of time.

The pitfalls of memory consolidation bring to mind the experience of a teenager diagnosed with mild FASD. A few hours after attending a parent-teacher meeting with his adoptive mother, he could not talk. Reflecting similar emotional experiences, foster moms' have stated that adolescents need "medications just to keep up, just trying to be normal." The chemical processes in neurons may not hold up when confronted with the demands of emotional information processing, in a brain with structural and possible neurochemical damage. Thus, cognitive deficits may emerge when damaged reorganized neural systems are unable to respond appropriately, particularly under stressful and environmentally challenging circumstances (Spear et al. 2002).

This memory consolidation theory, also called cellular consolidation theory, now has been expanded to include "reconsolidation." Once a memory is reactivated, it returns to a labile state, reconsolidation then incorporates the new learning and undergoes the same time dependent memory process similar to that seen after the original learning (Nader, 2003). The textbook account of consolidated memory is that of a robust memory, resistant to interference. Yet, new research is emerging that upon memory activation in retrieval, the trace may reconsolidate. Although much of this research is focused on "false memory" relevant in legal cases, it adds to understanding consolidation: comparing and integrating new information with old.

Neurobiology of Learning

The biological basis of learning and memory: how the brain perceives, stores, and retrieves memories, was first explored in depth by Lashley and later by Hebb. Lashley's classic work found that memory is widely distributed throughout large regions of the brain, localized in multiple sites distributed among the neurons. Lashley's results are consistent with the idea of having many kinds of sensory information: for example, visual, spatial, and olfactory separately processed and localized (Squire 1986).

Brain anatomy and brain chemistry are changed, at the level of the neuron, by learning. Hebb's synaptic theory looked at physiological properties of the nervous system. He proposed that, because neurons of similar function are grouped together, memory-traces were located in *cell assemblies*, groups of neurons with synaptic connections. According to Hebb, a cell assembly is formed and connections developed by learning and experience. Excitation of any neuron in the assembly activates the entire assembly. Memories are stored in these cell assemblies; thus, a memory can be stored and retrieved by any sensation: sights, sounds, smells, tastes, touch, thoughts, or emotions that activate some of the neurons in the cell assembly (Bloom and Lazerson 1988; Gregory 1989). Hebb proposed that synaptic connections become stronger when two interconnected neurons fire at the same time (Hebb 1949). "The modern view is that memory is widely distributed but that different areas store different aspects of the whole" (Squire and Kandel 1999). Specific regions have specialized functions which contribute to the storage of memories. Prenatal damage effects the potential of these connections.

Crick and Koch (2003), have provided a framework to understand the dynamics of neuronal coalitions; explanations, that expand Hebb's cell assembly theory. Detection of sensory input is not just a simple correlation, but a complex detection of correlations among other areas. For example, visual information is often incomplete, the cortical networks fill-in make their best guess. Many excitatory and inhibitory neurons act by forming temporary coalitions. They also speculate that the chemical internal dynamics of the neuron might affect the strength of coalitions: influencing what is required for information to reach consciousness. Coalitions form, grow or disappear.

Memory–Emotion Strengthens

Memory consolidation of experiences accompanied by emotionally arousing information is modulated in the amygdala (a part of the limbic system). Emotional memories have an added degree of strength and persist longer. In addition to memory consolidation for ordinary facts in the hippocampus, the amygdala may influence consolidation throughout the brain. Rats, with healthy brains, faced with tasks that require processing across different neural systems demonstrate that the amygdala promotes processing of multiple memory systems (McIntyre, Marriott, and Gold 2003).

Consistent with the importance of emotional content to memory is the hypothesis that the amygdala modulates long-term memory. Quevedo and colleagues (2003) found subjects given emotionally arousing material had a greater percentage of correct answers demonstrating, that emotional arousal enhanced long-term memory. Whereas studies have shown long-term memory is increased when the emotional content is arousing enough to be modulated by the amygdala; emotional intensity has not been found to influence short term or working memory.

The amygdala appears to serve to regulate the strength of explicit conscious declarative memories in relation to their emotional significance; hence contributing an emotional opinion. "Thus, the more active the amygdala at the time of learning, the more it enhanced the storage of those declarative memories that had emotional content" (Squire and Kandel 1999). In a supportive finding, Hamann's (2003) review of odors, found that the amygdala responded on the basis of emotional intensity, to both pleasant and unpleasant odors. Thus, arousal level contributes to the processing of an emotional experience.

Many modern day threats must be learned, for personal or family well-being. Morris, deBonis, and Dolan (2002) found an increase in neural responses in the amygdala to fearful facial expressions, and speculate that other structures (superior colliculus and posterior thalamus) were also implicated in processing the emotional information of fearful eyes.

The unconscious process of "priming" improves the speed and efficiency of perception for recently encountered stimuli, one more step in the early stages of memory (Squire and Kandel 1999). The unconscious attention to a stimuli cause us to respond with greater recognition each time new information is encountered.

Crick and Koch (2003) speculate that the firing of neuron coalitions influence the penumbra, the surrounding region. This penumbra filled with memories of past associations, expected consequences, movements, etcetera, may be a site of priming.

We recognize something unconsciously, possibly alerting associated areas; thus, preparing us with information, preparing us for action. Learning without concurrent awareness of what is being learned. Some responses to sensory inputs are rapid, transient and alert at an unconscious level. Once alerted, the brain then can work with a slower conscious system allowing time for thinking and planning.

Keep this in mind, as one piece of the possible explanations, when trying to understand the youngster with behaviors inappropriate to the situation. Emotional learning that developed unconsciously, without introspection, without awareness; may be asserting influence.

Long-Term / Short-Term - Working Memory

Ebbinghaus discovered that memories have different life spans. Some memories are short-lived and retained for minutes; others are long-lived and persist for days to months. Immediate memory lasts for seconds and holds five to seven items. Information in short-term memory, also called working memory, lasts minutes to a few days, just long enough to decide whether new material is worthy of being analyzed further, acted on, or stored in long-term memory. Alan Baddeley described "working memory" as requiring the simultaneous storage and processing of information: the control of attention, manipulation of visual information, and language (Baddeley 1992).

Immediate memory, that lasts only seconds, is reinforced by promptly asking the child to repeat what has just been heard. Short-term memory that lasts a few days is reinforced by asking questions after a delay of at least several minutes, a delay that is taken up by other activities (Rapin 1988). Long-term memory lasts days or even years as forgetting and reorganization of synaptic connections between neurons is stabilized (Squire & Kandel 1999).

Interference is a real detriment to learning for youngsters with neurologically damaged arousal systems, that have difficulty focusing and maintaining attention. Errors can occur at any point: encoding, storage, retrieval. Regarding focusing attention, "In short, the brain is designed to work most efficiently when it works on a single task and for sustained rather than intermittent and alternating periods of time" (Restak, 2003). Common external distractions divert attention: someone new enters a room, unsuspected movements, noises. Refocusing attention after a disruption is time-consuming, requiring a review of recently stored information. When interference is reduced, learning accuracy and speed improve. A fragmented attention focus may disrupt performance on immediate recall; impoverished learning or poor memory may also muddle recall performance. Use a learning strategy to side-step this.

Daniel Schacter (2001) in his book, *The Seven Sins of Memory*, details how memory can get the smartest person in trouble: transience, absentmindedness, blocking, misattribution, suggestibility, bias, and persistence. Transience, a sin of omission: is the loss of memory over time. Absentmindedness, a sin of omission: occurs when we do not focus on what we need to. Blocking, a sin of omission: is failure to retrieve a fact. Misattribution, a sin of commission: assigning a memory to the wrong source. Thinking something happened in one situation, when it happened in another. Suggestibility, a sin of commission: implanted memories resulting from leading questions or comments when a person is trying to remember. Bias, a sin of commission: revising a memory to make it fit ones current knowledge and beliefs. Persistence, repeated recall of emotionally disturbing information or events.

Keep in mind the seven sins when evaluating the story telling one often finds with youngsters who have FASD. Filling memory gaps with inappropriate words and confabulation, sorely tempts the listener to use truth telling as the judge; to fill the situation with right or wrong–good or bad motives. Memory monitoring deficits can contribute to memory distortions.

EXPLORING THE NATURE OF MEMORY RETRIEVAL

Retrieval of information is more successful when combined cues are utilized to produce recall. "If an initial single cue fails to facilitate a correct response, presenting a second cue coupled with the original first cue will be much more effective than presenting a different single cue" (Weidner and Jinks 1983). For example, if you asked "What is Alice's last name?" and the child couldn't remember, ask "What is Alice's last name? Her last name starts with the letter M." Partial learning and awareness of a small portion of the whole can trigger recall of the whole. The semantic flexibility of a single word cue can facilitate recall even though the word was not present in the original learning situation, directing the youngster to the appropriate memory. The same meaning was accessed by both word cues.

Information that is perceived and stored in several sensory and perceptual systems, that has a strong semantic component, is less subject to be forgotten. Recall is anchored in the way information was stored. Recall errors can occur because something was misperceived; perception errors rather than forgetting (Baddeley 1976). When using many cues you are more likely to find at least one cue that accesses a memory retrieval path (Baddeley 1982; Mishkin and Appenzeller 1987). For example, rather than using visual imagery; consider the possibility of using kinesthetic motor/movement, such as moving one's hand up and down as if bouncing a ball to retrieve information regarding basketball.

"If the cue is weak or ambiguous, what is reactivated might even differ from what was stored" (Squire and Kandel 1999). Is poor performance a reflection of a retrieval memory deficit or a storage memory deficit? Recognition memory lets one take advantage of partial learning. A single feature, possibly irrelevant, inadequate for complete recall may be sufficient for recognition of semantic, visual, and auditory interconnections (Hunt 1982; Alkon 1989). Using recognition tasks as part of learning practice, works like repetition to strength memory. Recall tends to increase the likelihood of subsequent recall.

Some things are easy to remember. A short poem is easier to memorize than a long one; an interesting story is easier to recall than a dull one. Youngsters understand and remember when the information is meaningful within the context of their experience and development.

Concrete objects that we can visualize are easier to remember than abstract words. We can look at six balls and recognize this amount without counting. With more balls, we often make mistakes. Our perceptual limitations are overcome by manipulating the available information: for example, counting by sets of two (Baddeley 1976).

State of Mind

Memory, retrieval of information, is enhanced when we are in the same physical, mental, and emotional state of mind we were in when learning occurred (Maguire 1990). Sad moods influence the memory of negative experiences. Happy mood states are associated with remembering positive experiences, higher memory performance, and use of faster more efficient information processing strategies (Forgas, Burnham, and Trimboli 1988; Squire and Kandel 1999). In addition, memory is likely to be modified by the current context in which information is retrieved (Aslin 1984). "Overall, retrieval is most successful when the context and the cues that were present when the material was first learned are the same as the context and the cues that are present later when making an attempt to recall" (Squire and Kandel 1999). For example, our perception of an orange is based on the visual features of shape and form, along with memories of our experiences with oranges, and the significance of an orange to us now.

> Develop cueing strategies for students who forget the words and directions before starting a task.

Sensory experiences that bring back memories of different senses are common. We have all experienced a voice on the telephone that prompts a visual memory of the caller's face. We remember things more efficiently when we are in a mood similar to the one we experienced during learning. For instance, the rehearsal atmosphere entertainers (actors, dancers) use: the stage, the music, the words, and the emotions, resemble the final performance environment.

Table 11. Memory Retrieval Tidbits.

- *Combined cues* facilitate recall.
- If an initial single cue fails to facilitate a correct response, *presenting a second cue coupled with the original first cue* will be much more effective than presenting a different single cue.
- Retrieval of a memory is enhanced when one is in *the same physical and emotional mood state* as in the original learning situation.
- Partial memories may be accessed using *recognition* activities.
- Cues with *meaningful associations* enhance recall.
- *Concrete objects* that we can visualize are easier to remember than abstract words.

(Baddeley 1976; Weidner and Jinks 1983; Mishkin and Appenzeller 1987)

Organization of Information

In addition to using sensory and perceptual systems, our minds make order out of experiences by grouping them in categories. These categories represent our theory about the characteristics of the objects in them, by noticing patterns and consistencies (Hunt 1982). Organized material is easier to learn, easier to remember. Most information about the world comes to us in a random order. We tend to create our own organization and meaning from this random stream of material (Baddeley 1982).

Youngsters with deficits in their ability to organize information, profit from curriculum design and the sequencing of instruction based on external organizational strategies. Youngsters that have been diagnosed as having attention deficit hyperactive disorder with a learning disability have difficulty processing and remembering a correct sequence of information (Kataria, Hall, Wong, and Keys 1992). Youngsters with FASD/FDE are likely to have similar deficits in the way incoming sensory/perceptual data is organized by the brain.

Repetition

Repetition turns a conscious voluntary act into an unconscious involuntary automatic act: into a habit, as skill develops the task is executed with ease and accuracy. Habits become sufficiently automatic, leaving attention free. The development of habits can be based on either noncognitive or cognitive systems. Noncognitive habits are automatic responses to a stimulus; such as holding a fork, knowing where the dishes go, recognizing when to clean the table. Cognitive habits are responses based on knowledge: such as spelling, and defining words (Mishkin and Appenzeller 1987). It takes time and practice to make a new habit permanent: structure, repetition, and consistency foster the development of habits.

Early studies on repetition by Ebbinghaus in 1885 give us a basis for understanding the effect of repetition on learning. Studies of repetition by Irvin Rock indicate that we form mental associations instantly. The role of repetition is to help us retain what we have already learned. Ebbinghaus concluded that "as the number of repetitions increase, the series are engraved more and more deeply and indelibly" (Schacter 1982). Repetitive practice distributed over time produces a stronger memory than many repetitions over a short time (Ebbinghaus 1964; Rock 1958). The use of repetition from presentation of information to recall: practice, practice, practice is a valuable tool.

Ebbinghaus found that retention of information increased when there were many repetitions in the original learning situation. Spaced and repetitive presentations of information enhance memory rather than massed training (Mattson and Roebuck 2002; Schacter 1982; Baddeley 1976; Ebbinghaus 1964; Rock 1958). Mattson and Roebuck (2002), found that the poor memory commonly reported in youngsters with FASD; reflects deficits in the initial amount of information learned, for verbal information. Repeated original learning trials allow more information than with only one presentation. Again in 2004, Mattson and Roebuck found that semantic information, meaning, aided recall. The suggestion here is to use learning strategies that provide opportunities to rehearse new information which include semantic information. Difficulty learning new information may impact reten-tion more than poor memory; given that the subjects with FASD, were as able as subjects without FASD to remember. Rather than reques-tioning the youngster that doesn't know an answer, reteach.

Table 12. Practice/Repetition.

I. We form mental associations instantly.

II. Repetition helps us RETAIN what we have already learned.

III. Curve of Forgetting: *most forgetting occurs during the first few hours after presentation.*
  A. Immediate feedback increases learning success.
  B. New information should be tested shortly after presentation to strengthen it.
    1. If correct: re-present information after a long delay (a few days).
    2. If in error: re-present information after a short delay (three minutes-one hour).

IV. *Present Many repetitions,* of significant information, in the original learning situation.

V. The *Amount of information* presented increases retention: elaboration of information to be learned makes it memorable.

VI. *Spaced presentations and spaced practice* enhance memory: repetitions distributed over time produce stronger memories than massed repetitions.
  A. Learning a single concept will require few presentations.
  B. Learning concepts that will generalize require a wide range of presentations and examples.
  C. Practice a new skill over a period time.

VII. Limitations of perception are overcome by *organizing/categorizing* the information avail-able.
  A. When asked to repeat three to six digits we can recall them correctly, when asked to recall fifteen digits we may remember less than two.
    1. If you have ten items, present these items two at a time.
    2. *Group digits rhythmically, by three's* or if not possible by three's, by two's and three's.

VIII. Intellectual *creativity is available after learning has occurred,* providing an opportunity for continued learning based on problem solving, using understanding and thinking.
  A. Children make about twice as many comments on stories that are familiar to them.

Ebbinghaus 1964; Rock 1958; Martinez and Roser 1985; Schacter 1982; Baddeley 1976)

In agreement that it looks like a memory problem, but is a prob-lem with the original learning: Kaemingk, Mulvaney, and Halverson (2003) found after four presentations, the FAS/FAE group retained information no differently than the controls when asked to recall 13 to 16 words, and learning 12 to 14 visual-spatial locations of designs. "We can arrange for multiple learning episodes instead of just one, we can rehearse the material to ourselves, and we can build into the learning context retrieval cues that will likely be present when memory is later to be used" (Squire and Kandel 1999).

Ebbinghaus is also famous for his Curve of Forgetting, which shows that most forgetting occurs during the first few hours after presentation of information and decreases thereafter (Ebbinghaus 1964; Schacter 1982). Testing new information shortly after its presentation will strengthen it. If the learner makes an error, the information should be re-presented after a short delay (three minutes - sixty minutes). If the learner is correct the material should be re-presented after a long delay (a few days).

Both Irvin Rock and Ebbinghaus found that the amount of information presented influences retention. For example, when asked to repeat three digits we can recall them correctly, but when asked to recall fifteen digits we may remember less than two. If you have ten items to present, give them two at a time. Group digits rhythmically, by three's or if not possible by three's, by two's and three's.

Introducing new information in small parts, allowing for mastery of each part before additional material is introduced provides the practice some students need. Students presented with new words that built on an existing base of knowledge, spent one-third the time necessary for skill mastery than students rapidly introduced to the new material. Specifically, after starting with a base of three words, students were not introduced to new words until all previously introduced words were learned (Gleason, Carnine, and Vala 1991). Curriculum materials may need to be supplemented with practice as few curriculum materials provide the amount of practice/repetition many students need.

Generalization

If a new task fits with what we have previously learned, our earlier learning can be transferred to the new situation. If not, the task is much harder to master. Events that are only moderately different, but still related to information we are familiar with, elicit a longer span of attention than either familiar information or novel events (Kagan 1972). Prior training transfers to the learning of a similar task, as with the students learning new words. An inability to generalize information from one situation to another can be compensated for by giving instructions in the environment skills will be used: the same location, the same time, the same mood state.

Learning a single concept requires only a little information and a few presentations. Learning complex concepts that generalize to many situations need a broad fund of information in the original learning situation, along with later presentations of additional information. Elaboration of information to be learned promotes the likelihood of retention and effective memory retrieval.

Redundancy and Predictability

The redundancy of language increases comprehension. English sentences are about 75 percent redundant. When we read or listen, all our knowledge of word meaning and grammar come to our aid. Semantic plausibility, grammatical complexity and length, in addition to word meaning influence comprehension (Kudo 1984). Semantically congruent, probable sentences are more comprehensible than improbable sentences. The unfamiliar is difficult to understand and remember correctly. Present new information in language your students understand.

Word recognition is superior for syntactically and semantically organized sentences, than incomplete sentences. For instance, we try and finish incomplete sentences, like finding a puzzle piece we check our fund of definitions. Using comprehension as a focus for teaching reading will take advantage of the fact that "recognition of words in sentences is superior to recognition of words in isolation" (Wright and Garrett 1984). Sentence structure and word meaning interact as reading combines the process of word recognition with the process of syntactic organization and semantic interpretation. Reading instruction that includes comprehension skill activities makes use of this natural predisposition. We tend to create a meaningful structure from unrelated words. Better comprehension equals better recall.

Reading

The processes underlying many academic tasks, such as reading, while available to the normal child, may be absent or inefficient for the youngster with FASD/FDE. Reading is composed of a number of processes: auditory sequencing, visual-motor-spatial integration, auditory and visual integration, along with demands on short-term memory. A deficit causing the breakdown of any single process results in reading difficulties (White and Miller 1983; Aaron 1981). For example, difficulty with syntax impacts both verbal and written expressive language. Deficits related to the types of information contained in reading material (graphic, orthographic, semantic, syntactic, and phonological) may be related to kindred language disorders, as they correspond with major components of language.

Dyslexia, reading problems not based on comprehension, but based on grasping the association between letters and phonemes, can be reversed after phonologic processing and decoding reading intervention. Dyslexia can be comorbid with other conditions. But, based on fMRI findings, looking at the brain reading, dyslexia is beginning to be understood as a variation on normal brain development rather than brain damage, impaired phonological processing that can be remediated with instruction that makes the rules of phonics clear (Shaywitz and Shaywitz 2003). Systematic phonics instruction beginning with the simplest patterns, and rules for all the ways to spell each of the approximately 40 phonemes for English is effective in improving reading decoding, fluency, and comprehension: learning how letters represent the sounds of words in reading. Infants that are shown pictures in a book and read aloud to as soon as they are born, who are read to daily, are more likely to become good readers.

Thinking and Creativity

The value of repetition extends to the intellectual creativity available after learning has occurred, providing an opportunity for continued learning and problem solving. The overlearning produced by repetition facilitates the development of understanding and thinking.

Examples of intellectual creativity based on knowledge of how the social and physical world works are found in early reading activities. When reading literature, children made about twice as many comments about familiar stories they had read many times. Children asked more questions when a story was unfamiliar and made more comments when a story was familiar (Martinez and Roser 1985). Knowledge makes us better problem solvers. As learners gain new insight into a topic, performance significantly improves.

Intellectual exploration requires an existing knowledge base to examine, reformulate, and construct new ideas. Once familiarity is achieved, verbal and written expression based on thinking about and organizing thoughts is possible (Roit and McKenzie 1985). Knowledge is used to make inferences, to answer questions, to guide thought processes, and to keep behaviors consistent with the existing situation: the goal of learning.

Development Influences Learning

Maturity changes the choice and complexity of information we remember; thus, the presentation of information and questions used must be adjusted. The growing developing child is in the process of transforming at each moment. Development changes the selection of what can be attended to and what attention choices are made. Infants learn different things than adults do about an experience. The complexity of information that can be processed at different ages changes; information that was learned at an earlier age may appear different to a more mature system (Aslin 1984). Nonverbal information such as smell, touch, and motor responses, are the foundation of an infant's knowledge. Words replace these nonverbal memories. Increasing maturity and new experiences result in a constant renewal of information. The strategies and cues one uses to successfully remember information change with development and maturity.

Developmental milestones indicate when a specific skill normally emerges and when it can be mastered. Given a supportive environment, a normally developing child acquires skills according to an orderly progression of difficulty.

Developmental delays result from disturbances to this maturation process. Deficits indicate subtle organic brain pathology rather than delayed maturation. Children with developmental delays improve with age, but children that have damaged brains do not just catch up. When a child's system is not intact, there are likely to be skill acquisition differences outside of what is typical (Kagan 1972). Development alone will not ameliorate damage. "The evidence today is that in many if not all children the 'developmental' disorders of higher cortical function reflect subtle organic brain pathology rather than delayed maturation" (Rapin 1988). To complicate the assessment and instruction picture, youngsters with deficits are likely to also have developmental delays (Aaron 1981). O'Malley (2003) adds ". . . not all developmentally disabled youth are mentally retarded, although all mentally retarded youth are developmentally disabled."

An aspect of attributing learning problems to maturational lag is the resulting ineffective instructional strategies. In error, developmental delays, which improve with age, are addressed rather than using strategies to compensate deficits that persist. When dealing with a deficit, instructors have to watch how students respond, and teach to the students learning style and strengths; side stepping deficits and eliminating instruction that require a missing capability. For example, if information is presented verbally to someone who is better at remembering visual information, learning will not be as robust. When looking at the youngster with FASD/FDE, developmental deficits require instructional strategies that focus on strengths as opposed to the developmental delays that are corrected by practice and maturation.

Each child has a unique pattern and timing of growth and development: the youngster with a normal brain will learn differently than the youngster with a damaged brain. Acceptance is the first step to fit adult expectations to a child's capabilities and range of social and intellectual skills. Children who have deficits can learn new skills using remedial strategies and interventions that circumvent deficits; teaching to strengths. Base the choice of intervention strategies on whether deficiencies are permanent or develop with age.

Chapter 7

COMMUNICATION

How efficient we are at expressing ourselves and understanding others, by speech, writing, reading, or gestures, influence how effective we will be throughout all aspects of our lives. Spoken language and gestures learned as a young person interacts with people in the environment, is ongoing continuously adjusting and refining throughout one's life.

Medical research on youngsters prenatally drug exposed is based primarily on children younger than school age (up to ten years), and youngsters with FASD/FDE are seldom specified in the speech/language research. Despite these limitations a variety of speech/language deficiencies found in the population of youngsters receiving special education services, along with remedial techniques are discussed in this chapter.

As a result of language or speech deficits, behavior can take on more communication functions of the broad mix of skills we bring to a situation. The options available when responding to new and common situations are based on the range of one's verbal and nonverbal communication skills. If you have ten behavioral options you can bring to a situation, your life will be more manageable then if you only have two. For instance, screaming or compliance; learning to communicate effectively improves the quality of one's social interactions.

LANGUAGE

Noam Chomsky theorized that language is inherited, not learned, and we are born predisposed to language, discovering rules for combining sounds into words. Children unconsciously master most of the grammatical rules of language by age six. We understand and produce sentences never before encountered. We learn how to combine words into sentences and take turns in conversation. Chomsky viewed linguistics as a theory about the functioning of the human mind (Moskowitz 1978; Crain 1980; Chomsky 1986; Pinker 2000). Infants recognize all phonemes, the individual sounds of a language. Within a year the child becomes increasingly able to differentiate only those phonemes commonly used by parents, and begins to lose the ability to perceive other phonemes. Recognition of parents speech sounds becomes primary to language development. Remember using baby talk, motherese? You modified your speech and word choices in terms of a baby's grammar and understanding. Motherese helps babies learn the specific sounds of language by making the sound structure very clear, keeping sentences shorter and simpler and by liberal use of repetition (Gopnik et al. 1999).

Speech requires precise coordination of lips, tongue, and breathing to change quickly from one sound to another to produce a word. Children usually make the following consonant sounds in babbling, and vocal play: b, m, p, d, t, n, g, k, w, h, f, v, th, s, z, l, and r. The first consonant sounds used are typically b, m, and p; called bilabials: meaning the child needs to use both lips to produce them, the lip smacking sounds you hear during feeding, the "m" sound during sobbing.

The lexicon of a language, the vocabulary of a language including morphological and syntactic information, is both an expression of culture and a part of it; providing a structure with which to frame communication and understanding.

LANGUAGE DEFICITS

Some youngsters have language disorders that are overshadowed by poor speech, poor hearing, or problems with perseveration and sequencing. Susceptible to the effects of interference, information may become cluttered with irrelevant facts, jeopardizing many aspects of learning. Academic success, particularly reading and writing reflect early language development. As the first step in the development of reading is understanding that written spellings represent the sounds of spoken words.

Youngster's verbal and nonverbal skills may be atypical: youngsters may fail to speak certain words, or err in the use of function words such as pronouns and conjunctions, or form words improperly, or make word choice substitutions related to semantically interchangeable meanings. The processing of speech sounds: the acoustic analyses of a word the youngster hears can be impaired. It can look like comprehension is limited when auditory information is insufficient.

Typical language development is sequential. Children who are not acquiring language according to a normal pattern may not be developing with this systematic sequential progression of skills. In fact, for children with deficits, the progression of developmental language milestones may be deviant. Language disordered children have less in common with children developing normal language patterns than with other language disordered children (Arwood 1983).

Young children with FASD/FDE may just observe rather than use language to communicate, may prolong the use of infantile articulation, or not use language to communicate feelings, wants and needs. Ask them a question, they may answer off topic, or if *echolalic*, repeat the question back to you. They may use one and two-word sentences. Poor articulation is worsened by youngsters who make unusual sounds or use unusual pitch and loudness. With a lack of social awareness, they may inappropriately initiate interaction. For example, aggressive communication and negative interaction with peers: hitting, pushing, biting, swearing, negative remarks, or screaming.

Carney and Chermak (1991) compared the expressive and receptive language abilities of American Indian children developing normally and with FAS, using the Test of Language Development (TOLD). Older children with FAS were found to have syntactic deficits while younger children had more global language deficits. In interpreting their results they concluded ". . . it is unclear whether FAS causes language deficits or whether language deficits are but one of a cluster of symptoms resulting from depressed cognitive function" (Carney et al. 1991). Superficial verbal behaviors with limited content are found across all levels of FASD.

There are a variety of *aphasias*, language difficulties that reflect degrees of speech disruption. Two predominant types of aphasia are Broca's aphasia, resulting in poor articulation, and Wernicke's aphasia, resulting in poor comprehension. Paul Broca discovered a speech center in the brain responsible for the motor act of producing language. In Broca's aphasia speech is poorly articulated and effortful, but comprehension is unimpaired. Individuals realize they are not able to say words clearly. Carl Wernicke, discovered a center in the brain that is responsible for comprehension and formulation of spoken and written language. In Wernicke's aphasia, comprehension is poor, while speech is normally articulated, yet meaningless. Individuals are unaware their fluently articulated speech is incomprehensible.

Table 13. Language Development Deficits.

- Prolonged infantile articulation
- Prolonged nonverbal prelanguage
- Delayed acquisition of words, delayed semantic development
- Fewer spontaneous vocalizations from early infancy
- Poor comprehension
- Meaningless speech
- Nonverbal behavior inconsistent with verbal communication
- Impoverished use of words and gestures to communicate wants and needs.
- Communication does not show relationships as much as preferences, nonmeaningful preferences.

It is important for teachers, and other children to allow sufficient time for the student to respond in conversation. For example, Johnny has minor neurological damage that results in a very slow expressive language response time. Conversation requires the student to organize and select relevant information. He can answer questions and contribute, but impatient peers and adults frequently respond to his delayed response as if it were a conversational pause; as an opportunity to add to what the speaker is saying and add to the discussion, without waiting for Johnny's contribution. Some youngsters need more time to rehearse, to develop a response: impatience can suppress the development of their verbal communication responses. Allow the student time to finish, then paraphrase, making sure you the listener understand, as well as allowing the speaker one more chance to scrutinize the content of their communication.

How fast a speaker talks can affect the listener's ability to understand. If the presentation rate is too slow, attention wanders, if too fast the listener is overloaded. Remember some students are prone to articulate words slowly. Both articulation and comprehension may be slow. If speaking is slow and labored, listening may also be.

CONVERSATION AND EMOTIONAL TONE

Beyond word choice and grammar, vocal affect identifies expressions of emotion. Affective prosody, expressing and understanding the emotional content of language has been shown to be damaged in adults with FASD, who did not have overt aphasic deficits: the acoustic features of language that express emotion and attitudes, such as: rhythm, melody, pitch, pausing, intonation (Monnot, Lovallo, Nixon, and Ross 2002). Some voice tones put others off even before a social behavior can be evaluated and responded to. Speech and language therapists recommend voice training to make the voice "sound" normal: the rate at which a youngster speaks, pronunciation, speech rhythms, in addition to intonation of individual words and the entire sentence. Imitating environmental sounds, sound play is a recommended first step. For example, a school bus, wind on a windy day, a telephone ringing, etc. Next, to hold a listeners attention, after learning to vary one's voice, vary: posture, gestures, and location.

TEACHING STRATEGIES
FOR COMMUNICATION BEHAVIORS

Children with language disorders may not be able to effectively handle instructions or directions that are more than one or two concepts in length or complexity. Unable to process an instruction, a child can appear to be noncompliant. Consider, whether there are deficits in the underlying processes required to understand or execute a direction. Are there problems with auditory integration, with visual-motor-spatial integration, with the ability to coordinate perceptions with thinking comprehension processes? The relationships involved in a sequence of directions may not be understood. For example, a direction may have secondary instructions embedded within it that increase the complexity. (1) Go to [action] the big [size] red [color] cupboard [object]. (2) Take out [action] the little [size] can [object] of soup [food]. The complexity of this direction could be simplified by reducing the number of internal directions. To make sure the directions have been understood, ask the child to restate the directions. A youngster that doesn't understand what you want won't know how to respond.

Billie McKenzie, who has taken care of her fifteen-year-old grandson, Jamal, exposed to heroin in the womb since his birth; has found a successful strategy to compensate for his poor memory. She gives "one command at a time," Jamal is able to follow one command. This keeps Billie from getting upset with this child, who may appear non-compliant because the last two in a series of three directions have been forgotten. This is a highly effective technique, used by classroom teachers, speech clinicians as well as parents. It's easily taught and has immediate success.

Youngsters may be unable to keep up with the conversation, or follow directions because of a poor auditory memory. Remember, the infants with FDE that were easily overstimulated used avoidance, including auditory avoidance, to reduce stimulation. They also were limiting the development of their auditory memory. Improvement can be made by having students practice following instructions and repeating sentences that gradually increase in length and complexity. For example, increase the number of words in sentences the student is asked to repeat, one additional word at a time. Keep directions simple, clear, and specific. For example, say, "hold your spoon," rather that "hold it." A medical foster mom has found using concrete instructions and repeating instructions often, result in a greater likelihood that children will learn and complete tasks. She begins with a simple one-step direction: then she increases the number of steps, one step at a time, gradually increasing the number of directions. Giving instructions that require understanding more concepts than youngsters are familiar with contribute to failure.

Take advantage of opportunities to model language use by identifying and describing ongoing activities. For example, "Johnny is painting a green tree," or "I am putting the paints away now." Mary Berson, a classroom teacher, has found that "everything needs to be labeled." She states what students are going to do, "we are going to read from level one now," and asks students to verbally repeat descriptions of the classroom activities, "what are we going to do?"

Everyday life provides opportunities to develop the social aspects of language. Educators can identify and model use of words to appropriately express the child's interests and those of others. There is a serious social disconnect when the expressions of language and behavior do not fit together: model the behaviors that fit what is being said. Children with severe language problems demonstrate both consistencies and inconsistencies between nonverbal and verbal communication. For example, Jimmy asks to play with the ball, then drops it and runs off. Jimmy tells you he's hungry and wants to go to lunch, then doesn't eat. Keep in mind, youngsters that do not communicate feelings, wants, and needs may not understand what they feel, want, and need.

Attention to a broad range of verbal and nonverbal communication methods may be necessary. For example, a child's behavior is part of his/her language: crying, laughing, screaming, whining, moving, physical manipulation, pointing, eye gaze, directional reaches, signs, gestures. Reconceptualize behavior as communication, particularly with infants and youngsters who are less responsive, less clear, less interpretable in their cues. Focusing on the communication intent rather than language will uncover the most creative instructional strategies. Interact more, resist the normal human impulse to adapt to a child's low responsiveness, become **more** engaged. Encourage nonverbal communication for the expression of basic concepts and every day activities, particularly for the prelanguage or nonverbal child. Ordinary daily activities such as self-care and eating, provide opportunities to integrate intellectual with social communication skills.

Sign Language: American Sign Language (ASL) provides a gestural language communication tool for people with limited hearing or verbal abilities. Each sign represents a word. Signs that explain a situation are followed by the result; the most concrete or important element comes first, followed by adjectives, adverbs, or verbs. The word order in ASL is different from that in English, and combining ASL with verbal expressions offers optimal communication tools for some youngsters. Teaching a few basic signs (more, juice, change diaper, etc.) to all pre-language infants jump-starts communication.

COMMUNICATION BARRIERS

Barriers to effective communication can be emotional, mental or physiological. Physically, can the youngster hear and see, is a damaged perceptual system presenting an incorrect perspective, is the room too cold, is the lighting poor, is the background noise distracting? Internal as well as external distractions enhance or hinder communication.

Often incorrect beliefs form a barrier to good communication. We react emotionally to our thoughts and beliefs about an event and our actions correspond to those beliefs. Both you and the youngster bring your own fund of knowledge, physical and emotional background to a subject. For example, you believe that a youngster is malicious, but the youngster is scared; hence the belief is incorrect. Children who express what seems like angry behavior may be sad, afraid, or frustrated by an inability to communicate their needs. The youngster may think you're angry when you are just impatient and in a hurry. What factors are influencing communication?

Youngsters with FASD/FDE that are normal looking and use a broad vocabulary often confuse our expectations. The cues we need to accurately modify our speech when communicating with these youngsters are harder for us to detect. Despite an apparent verbal fluency some of these youngsters, particularly the older ones with some language skills, have communication that reflects a lack of comprehension. Possibly to divert attention they may use emotionally loaded words that stop communication: attacking, negative, malicious words. They may use excessive why questions and commands permeated with sarcasm: poor choices.

When we come under stress due to a child's negative behavior, our brain tends to shut down. We would do well to ignore communication that creates barriers. We cannot take it personally; we cannot respond in kind. Neg-ative verbal communication, like other negative behaviors, responds well to redirection: change the subject. Model a successful interaction by requesting a response from another student. Preserve self-esteem for everyone in the situation.

CONVERSATION STRATEGIES

Conversation is our most commonly used successful instructional strategy. Rules of conversation, *Pragmatics*, include: (1) speaking clearly (2) attending to, looking at, and listening to the speaker, (3) staying on the topic, and knowing when it's OK to change topics, (4) how to ask and answer questions. Involving children in conversation is the most natural way to help them learn these rules. Conversational interactions assist correcting a child's language errors because it follows the natural process of language acquisition, and supports the child's social needs for using language. Particularly in nondirective activities, use conversation rather than directions, commands, or asking questions. A student-teacher interactive conversational approach increases the likelihood of correctly understanding information, reducing the student's opportunity to learn incorrect information or incorrect responses. Moderately effected youngsters particularly, benefit less from adult correction (or criticism) of their errors than from discussion. Communication activities that foster comprehension include: summarizing, clarifying, questioning, and predicting outcomes.

Avoid continually asking, "what's this? "what's that?" Children need lots of experience and practice before they can respond successfully to questions. Demonstrate how to answer questions by asking yourself and answering your own questions aloud in front of the child. Model how questions are answered, remembering to model combining eye contact with communication: "what's that? . . . a dog . . . a furry dog" and then give the child time to respond or react. Ask simple "what, when, who, and how questions in the natural context of daily activities, e.g., "what's in the box?, where is your new toy?"

If possible, ask questions that encourage elaboration. Use of *open-ended questions* encourage descriptive responses rather than "yes," or "no." For example, "I wonder what you could do with this ball." By answering questions, the child learns to look for and select information, to paraphrase concepts, and to use examples. Questions encourage youngsters to formulate and elaborate an explanation.

Table 14. Language Development Activities.

Descriptive Talk - Child Centered: Describe what a child is doing, touching or seeing during everyday activities. For example, if a child is petting a cat, you can say: "you're playing with the cat, you're petting the cat, I can hear the big white cat purring." It is important to gear your Descriptive Talk to the level a child can understand. Keep sentences simple. Use a long enough conversational pause to give the child ample opportunity to respond. Use repetition generously repeating words as you talk; and to make repetition more effective, vary the tone of your voice, keeping in mind, voice tone indicates intensity, e.g., "you want a cookie, right now!"

Descriptive Talk - Adult Centered: Talking about what you are doing while the child watches helps a child attach words to activities and objects. For example, as you wash your hands, you can say: "I'm washing my hands, washing my hands with soap and water."

Descriptive Talk - Object Centered: Provide vocabulary for objects the child is using, touching, or seeing. For example, "It's a ball." "It's a big, red ball."

Expansion - Repeat and Add: Repeat what the child is saying and add more detail. For example: if the child says "cold" the adult can say "Yes, the snowball is cold." "The white snowball is cold."

PART III

Chapter 8

INSTRUCTION

This chapter presents instructional strategies teachers and other service providers of youngsters with FASD/FDE and related disorders have found effective for youngsters with inconsistent attention and/or poor utilization of learning strategies that need to learn how to learn. Interviews play an important part in this section providing examples of successful techniques using the external information processing strategies of structure, repetition, and consistency, including examples of presentation of information to multiple sensory pathways, and the use of concrete experiences.

Research on learning from studies of FASD/FDE and other disabilities provide guidance for meeting the social and educational needs of students with comparable damage. In order to pinpoint specific skills measured by a study, a narrow focus is essential; thus, researchers have used simpler tasks than the average learning situation demands, making extrapolating learning techniques limited. Adapting the complexities of each learning task to the aspects of a students preserved abilities, is the educator's clear focus.

Damaged mental processes interfere with the learning of normal tasks, a poor memory transfers little previous learning to a new task. The cognitive processes normally used to merge information from multiple sources, evaluate and organize it as a basis of action, if damaged, can be replaced with structure, repetition, and consistency: compelling actions to become based on habit and external organization. First, to determine which strategies will be effective, you have to recognize what characteristics are amenable to change. What is appropriate for one can be very wrong for another: follow the student's temperament and abilities. Choose instructional strategies that are related to the cognitive processes of individual learners, their personality, learning style, and development. Capitalizing on a youngster's strengths augments weaker areas in addition to developing strengths. Finding an instructional strategy that addresses the students strengths reduces the cumulative deficiencies resulting from a reliance on compensatory strategies alone.

Frequently evaluate the instructional strategies used, especially when teaching to a weakness as success can be compromised by the amount of damage to the specific brain areas needed for a task. When the student fails to complete a task, change the instruction: don't assume the student was not listening or paying attention: re-teach.

> If I am frustrated, I may give up trying.

An adult with FASD used "rules" to manage social situations. Recognizing his socially engaging personality was part of the behavioral characteristics of FASD, not everyone welcomes, his rule was "no talking first." Despite wanting to go up to and talk to everyone, this rule kept him from putting others off. When people who knew him approached and started talking, *then* it was okay for him to talk.

Role-play ways to ask for help and identify people who can help. My personal experience of this was a young lady who waited by the open classroom door at Portland State University for me to finish and let my students out for a break. She needed someone to help her find the bus stop, as street construction made it difficult for her to determine where the buses would stop. Maybe a graduate student taught her how to find a safe person to help, and how to wait in a calm, nonintrusive way. My whole class was impressed with her social grace and independent living skills.

INFORMATION PROCESSING STRATEGIES

Information processing strategies vary from one learner and one task to another. The effectiveness of strategies employed depends on the cognitive ability of the student and the complexity of the task. Any of several aspects of the learning task will influence which strategy can most enhance retention. A student who applies strategies that are inappropriate to the learning task is less effective than a student who spontaneously, or with prompting, applies task-appropriate processing strategies. Youngsters with FASD/FDE who have cognitive deficits, bring to a new task few, atypical, or at best fragmented information processing strategies.

Youngsters with FASD/FDE need instruction that is based on a detailed analysis of the specific learning task they are to master and their learning style. Students involved in training programs that have instruction based on learning style strategies, that include specific steps of a task broken down and sequentially presented, show enhanced performance (McDaniel and Kearney 1984). There are large individual differences in the kinds of strategies needed. Utilize the sensory preferences, sensory combinations and instructional techniques which are found to be the most effective for each individual student (Weidner and Jinks 1983).

The neurobiology of learning and memory support accessing many sensory pathways, particularly for the youngster with a unique learning profile. A *multisensory instructional approach* uses presentation of information to more than one of the primary senses: vision, olfactory, kinesthetic, tactile, and auditory. Accessing many sensory modalities takes advantage of all possible neurological pathways, providing instruction that addresses a learner's sensory strengths. These multiple sensory information pieces are coordinated into integrated perceptions. One medical foster mom found sentence writing helps her youngster remember, the action of writing accessed tactile and kinesthetic sensory strengths. Having youngsters apply all their senses can improve the execution of a task. Instructional strategies that rely on only **one** modality may exacerbate deficits, particularly when the instruction inadvertently focuses on a learner's weakness. Connect a weak area with a strong one. For example, present information combining a weak auditory sense with a strong visual sense.

Table 15. Information Processing Strategies.

Structure
Repetition
Consistency

Structure

Student's who do not have efficient strategies to understand and acquire information, who are unable to produce information processing strategies automatically, need to learn problem solving and memory strategies: most importantly, structure, repetition, and consistency. Techniques that consistently develop habits and information-processing strategies that follow them throughout life is a resource to be consistently drawn upon in all future learning situations.

> Learning to Learn = Information
> Processing Strategies.

Scheduling and organizing the day helps youngsters anticipate what will come next. Begin with structure, if students come to class and find materials on their desks, they can become actively involved right away. Rely on a ritual rather than on their internal organization. Keeping students engaged gives teachers the freedom to handle problems as they prepare to transition into the school day.

Youngsters with particularly limited cognitive flexibility, ineffectual organizational skills, poor memory, and limited verbal skills need external organizational tools. Schedules using verbal instructions with pictures, for example, directing a student to each activity using a "laminated photograph" of that student engaged in the activity (art, music, lunch, rest room, recess, reading, math), has been successfully used to help students' understand what is expected.

A junior high teacher incorporates structure and routine into school schedules by having students design and use their own "job-cards" (individual daily schedules for themselves). They design their own card, drawing little pictures, symbols, or words for each activity. In addition to the activities, behavior reminders are included on their job-cards. Students accept written daily activity schedules without the confusion and reluctance that can accompany verbal directions. Students with poor memory and organizational skills that may have difficulty keeping track of what to do now and what to do next are more successful using a written or graphic daily schedule to organize themselves. Along with task-completion, progress can be recorded as children check off completed work. Kindergarten and first grade teachers use written schedules posted on the wall to help young students organize themselves. Organizing the day with consistent scheduling, together with limiting interruptions and outside intrusions, reduces classroom confusion and help students stay organized and stay on task.

Predictable routine transition times with a consistent beginning, middle, and end assist the smooth flow of activities. Teachers in the Los Angeles pilot program found routine important. "Among the lessons gleaned from the two-year-old project: routine is crucial. Abrupt transitions from one activity to another can be unsettling" (Trost 1989). Can you change your mind if the normally fluid way of solving problems is limited by mentally clumsy processes? Mary Berson, a classroom teacher, cautions teachers to realize that if children are very engaged in an activity "it's hard for them to quit." They may be unable to stop or let go of a preferred object or activity. Give warnings. They may need a longer time to complete a task and may not know when an activity is over, or a task is complete. Routinely alert children when an activity will soon be over. Mary recommends making transition time into an activity, in and of itself. Each transition follows the same ritual, with a beginning, middle, and end. She prepares for transitions with warnings: five minutes before clean up, two minutes, thirty seconds; using concrete signals like the familiar, turning lights on and off. A transition activity, for example, could be to sing a song before starting the next activity. In a classroom serving disabled youngsters, I have successfully used a simple spelling activity for both transition and to fill unscheduled time gaps of under ten minutes. I would sound out a word, say the word, sound it out again, then have the students write it down. Classroom management at transition time demands that teachers are organized, prepared, and have materials ready. Organization must be external: youngsters cannot be expected to constructively use any free time between activities or quietly wait.

Repetition

Repetitive routines provide continuity and reliability. For example, schedule the beginning of reading instruction at the same time each day and have students sit in the same chair. Follow a sequence when presenting reading instruction: review sounds, learn new sounds, review known words, learn new words, discuss word meaning, then read a story. Repetitive routines and rituals provide memory jogger cues that help youngsters organize and manage their activities. Structuring the presentation of information in a consistent repetitive way helps provide the student with a strategy for organizing, understanding and remembering information. Ritual provides the "cueing" necessary to refocus attention.

Enlist the child's unique behaviors to develop rituals. For example, a second grade boy who slowly places his pencils, erasers, and crayons back in a specific order after each activity. A teacher's first response may be to discourage what looks like time-wasting behavior. Yet, encouraging him to use his innate ritual style to organize himself will help him develop a routine ritual style he can use in a variety of school/classroom situations to facilitate the successful adjustment between special services and the traditional classroom, encouraged by inclusion programs. A creative approach to the use of unique behaviors can produce successful results. Rituals and routines help youngsters feel organized and secure.

Consistency

Predictability and order strengthen a child's self-control, sense of security, and mastery over the environment. It helps students organize themselves in the classroom, if they have their own areas (their own shelves, desks, bulletin board space), and a consistent room arrangement (materials are right there, pencils are always in the same place, paints are always in the same place). Provide a predictable setting with continuity and reliability: children need to know where things are.

Youngsters can find a change in routine upsetting, making it difficult for them to learn. Having worked with youngsters who would get upset if activities were presented differently, teachers found consistency reduced disruptions and encouraged a smoother activity flow. They also recommend maintaining the flexibility to add more complex materials and ideas in response to a student's changing development within a structured consistent classroom. Consistency and routine work at home for Phyllis Williams, a medical foster mom, who recommends some freedom within established routines, the same dinner time, the same bedtime. "Polydrug kids seem to be able to function best with very narrow limits."

METHODS

The broad range of verbal and physical instructional methods teachers' have found useful include: *limited verbal* direction, telling students specifically what they need to know; *nonverbal cues*, activity pictures, physical gestures, and modeling; *demonstration*, showing children how to perform a task; *physical assistance*, helping children as they proceed through a task, guiding their hands, or the more direct hand over hand assist; *feedback*, telling children how they did or advising them to "do it this way." Whereas youngsters who demonstrate good comprehension of information commonly correct themselves when they make errors, the youngster with FASD/FDE often will not. Without feedback, these youngsters may practice their mistakes.

> Without feedback youngsters may practice mistakes.

Use concrete, verbal, and physical cues to direct or redirect the child. To alert her four-year-old student "Jim" with FDE, Robin Lindsley uses physical cueing, putting her hand on his shoulder signals transitions that require materials be put away. Soon other kids started helping Jim by putting their hand on his shoulder, modeling the teacher.

Beth Caruso combines verbal cueing with nonverbal physical cueing to enhance her communication, "the fewer words you use, the better off you are." Youngsters that do not persist with a task need techniques to focus and stay on task: some teachers rely on instructional statements, others on prompting statements, and others on reinforcing statements.

> "The fewer words you use, the better off you are"
> (Beth Caruso, prekindergarten teacher).

"*Self-instruction*," self-talk, verbalizing the steps of a task as each step of the task is executed, combines a memory retrieval tool with an organizational strategy. Provide verbal cues (talk the child through a task) if the child is unable to verbally give the steps of a task. A language instruction technique that combined self-instruction with teacher cueing was used successfully by Chris Amos, a prekindergarten teacher. Julie, with FDE, has a difficult time centering on a task, is easily distracted, and needs continuous cueing back to the task. Chris found routine, repetition, and verbal self-instruction a successful combination to teach her the order in which to carry out a series of steps. For example, teaching the sequence of tasks necessary for the execution of basic life skills; such as hanging up a coat or putting away school materials. Using self reminders, Julie said each step out loud, one at a time, when cued by the teacher: "tell me the next thing you will do." This prompting kept her on task and helped direct execution of the correct sequence. Even a weak association aids recall if it's presented during both the learning and recall situations. Verbally describing the steps of a task as the students perform a task can improve organization, learning speed and accuracy (Whitman, Spence, and Maxwell 1987). This very successful, simple to use, self-instruction technique provides the organization many youngsters need to complete a task.

Table 16. Instructional Adaptations.

It is the instruction, not the child, that must be modified

- Role-play "what will happen if" types of games for appropriate manners, and verbal responses.
- Add "happiness-inducing" activities.
- Provide two sets of books/workbooks—one for home and one for school use.
- Allow students a sufficient opportunity to explain their answers.
- Design worksheets/tests that allow students to answer in a response style they are comfortable with. For example, drawing pictures, cassette tapes, or videos.
- Students may like reading or composing stories into a tape recorder, or telling stories to other students.
- Class brainstorming to generate an extensive number of ideas or solutions to a problem by suspending criticism and evaluation.
- Extend testing/assignment time.
- Use communication boards or charts with pictures, symbols, numbers or words to express responses, and/or allow oral responses.
- Use lap desks or a table-top easel with cork that allows work to be attached with push pins, or tape.
- Improve grip for writing by placing rubber bands, rubber or plastic tubing around the shaft of the pen or pencil.
- Tie a pencil on a string to the desk for easier retrieval.
- Provide an audiotape of assignments and instruction/lectures.
- Pace verbal presentations to varying auditory comprehension rates.
- Provide written copies of board work.

- Use community-based lessons, with real-life events and concrete examples, have instruction and practice take place in the environment the skills and information will be used.
- Offer students a broad variety of actives that permit them to explore new skills and to practice previously acquired skills.
- Relate new learning to prior experience with specific examples.
- Corrective feedback Give a reexplanation, first using the same, then a different approach, then modeling the correct response.
- Give task specific feedback regarding the accuracy/inaccuracy of the student's responses.
- Use cooperative groups: partner learning, peer tutors, cross-age tutors.
- Replacement behavior: for example, perseveration can be stopped in many cases by changing a motor act. For example: John draws a circle over and over. The teachers says, "John give me your eraser" (a motor act), "now John draw a square" (a replacement behavior).
- Behavior caution: letting students have something when they ask in the wrong way (not using the skills student is working on).
- Face students with hearing impairments when speaking to them.
- Touching a student when he can *see you* is less disturbing. Unpredictable movements can be upsetting.
- Accompany verbal instruction with visual references and a demonstration.
- Wait a little longer than you think is necessary, give student extra time to analyze and execute the directions, to complete assignments.
- Direct communication to a youngsters ability level, for example, pointing according to fine motor abilities, e.g., pointing with fist, or tilting or nodding head toward a desired object, use a pencil as a pointer: point with the child's eye view.
- After a verbal explanation, model the expected behavior.
- Repeat directions as the student is doing the task.
- Have student repeat the directions prior to performing the task.
- Have student prove their understanding of directions by demonstrating the skills.
- Reteach, revisit important teaching points *often*.
- Using magnifiers for reading will enlarge the print, but the reading may be slower.
- Braille, because of the slowness of braille, allow the student more time to read an assignment.
- Daily assignments should be short and able to be accomplished within the scope of the student's abilities or with the aid of a support system.
- Encourage active participation by the student, limited passive listening.
- Encourage the student to ask questions, praising initiative.
- Teach the student to recopy, revise, and review class notes as *soon as possible* after class.
- Teach the students to date and kept class notes in an orderly system of notebooks or files.
- Keep folders of baseline work (e.g., samples of best handwriting) and ask the learner to compare his or her work with his or her "best "
- If the student has more than one teacher, coordinate instructional strategies and task completion standards.
- Provide objects or pictures to help the student stay on the topic.
- Use simplified vocabulary and provide a study sheet with terms or facts required to comprehend the subject.
- Highlight texts or worksheets to indicate critical information. Encourage students to high-

light–provide student with a school text that can be marked up.
- Condense lengthy directions into steps, i.e., 1–2–3.
- Have students make models, draw, or demonstrate relevant subject matter.
- Require fewer questions or problems to be completed for homework, seatwork, etc. (i.e., 5 math problems instead of 8).
- Allow student to take tests by having it read to her/him.
- Allow student to tape homework and reports instead of writing them.
- Use computation aids such as, special rulers, grids, graph paper, a calculator, etc.
- Use learning centers based on specific subjects with learning packets, or student-directed activities, for example, science materials and experiments.
- Physical organization of materials: subject level areas that contain shelves, drawers, and containers. For example, a handwriting section could have tracing stencils, and lined paper; things to be squeezed for development of hand strength.
- Student progress worksheets and progress graphs are motivational; providing a concrete skill acquisition reference.
- Use a system for checking off steps as they are completed.
- Use student contracts to clarify and make expectations concrete.
- Use communication: letters and notices to parents keep motivation up.
- Homework: train parents to use instructional strategies that are consistent with classroom strategies.
- Photograph students performing a task the correct way and use it as a concrete example.
- Laminate a duplicate of workbooks or worksheet pages that can be used over and over for practice.
- Leaving and returning to class management: have sign-out and sign-in sheets with space for the time, along with the hall passes.
- Behavior in line: minimize time expected to stand and wait.
- Behavior in line: avoid crowded or noisy hallways.
- Read favorite books again and again and again.
- Modifications for secondary and high school students: Substitution of courses or Waiver of courses.
- Invite learner feedback.

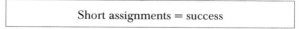

Short assignments = success

Adapted from the contributions of educators in my graduate courses, and Mann, P. H., Suiter, P. A., & McClung, R. M. (1992).

Multisensory Instructional Techniques

Multisensory instructional techniques that present information to multiple senses provide a strategy for the development of substitution tricks that circumvent damaged areas; thus, accessing a learners' strengths. Simultaneous sensory input, utilizing sensory combinations together with a consistent structured presentation, help learners reroute brain cell pathways to develop the most effective information processing strategies; even when the teacher isn't sure which sense is the strongest.

Presenting information to multiple senses allows the most functional modality to be used as a primary path for learning. When learning to read the word "cake," students can see the word, hear it spoken, write it, and discuss how a cake smells as it bakes. Instructional techniques directed at a student's sensory preference utilizing the strongest sensory combinations are found to be the most effective (Weidner and Jinks 1983). However, a multisensory instructional approach caution is needed: involving many sensory modalities may overwhelm the person who is hypersensitive to a specific sensory modality.

Generalization: Instruction in the Environment

Youngsters with FASD/FDE may have difficulty remembering the sorts of information required for everyday life. A medical foster mom tells of her son losing bicycles. When he arrives at a location, he parks his bike and gets busy with his new activity, forgetting where his bike is. His poor memory, combined with an inability to generalize information to the new situation, makes it necessary for him to learn a specific ritual that can be used every time he parks his bike so he can remember where it is. Memory deficits often accompany an inability to generalize and to transfer learning to new or novel situations. Phyllis Williams, a medical foster mom with an R.N. nursing background, finds she needs patience working with youngsters who can't remember, who can't apply information learned in one situation to another. "If you tell a child something 1,000 times and he still doesn't retain it, it takes great patience to say it 1,001 times. You have to consider it a bonus if he retains it." Phyllis finds structure and routine helpful techniques to circumvent memory deficits.

Instructions given in situations where skills are used help compensate for a limited ability to generalize. Carol, a special education teacher with many years of experience, takes her students to the local grocery store for a life-skills shopping lesson. This is a once a week activity to purchase food for the classes' daily snack. Her students have a list of items they are to find and as a group they take turns helping each other find items and then go through the checkout with Carol to purchase the groceries. Learning is integrated with experience for these students. Learning and using skills in a functional and meaningful context in the environment skills will be used.

A variety of skills have been learned and generalized by persons who are severely mentally handicapped. We can expect similar skill development from youngsters with FASD/FDE. Persons with mental handicaps can be taught to generalize skills and information to a variety of tasks: self-help, communication, street crossing, transportation, leisure activities, and vocational activities (Ferretti 1989). Children who can't generalize see every day as a new day–every minute as a new minute. An inability to generalize is often exacerbated by a poor memory. They can't generalize. They can't remember. From one day to the next aspects of academic, basic self-care, and social skills are lost. When generalization has failed to occur, the skills taught appear to be nonfunctional, restricted to the context in which the skills were learned. Memory is enhanced when the learning situation is in the same situation in which an individual needs to remember and use the skills: the same time, the same place, the same physiological state, the same emotional state of mind.

Perceptual, Motor, and Spatial Skills

Educators working in the school with students who have FASD/FDE find these youngsters have a variety of motor problems: abnormal reflexes, poor motor organization, poor quality muscle tone, disorganized motor activity, and difficulty performing integrated motor acts. Individuals with impaired motor skills need physical therapy to help with motor development: walking, crawling, swinging, climbing, throwing, catching, jumping, running and balancing. For example, a child may not have enough muscle tone to maintain an upright sitting position, and delayed gross motor abilities make it difficult to sit on a chair and attend. Make sure this student's physical position is stable enough so that he does not have to devote his whole attention to maintaining balance on the chair. Modeling and guiding large and small motor control development provide opportunities for integrating sensory-motor with spatial relationships, using objects that have a variety of spatial dimensions such as pegboards, puzzles, blocks, and outdoor games. Poor eye-hand coordination due to problems with muscle control in addition to difficulties with spatial perception, make eating neatly a challenge. The perceptual adaptation process involves maintaining normal coordination, while adjusting to and clarifying new sensory input. For example, adaptation during physical activity is stable, yet sufficiently modifiable to allow adaptation for changing circumstances. Running when the ground is wet, when it's raining versus when it's dry on a hot ninety degree day, we run slightly differently on wet ground than we do on hot, dry ground. Problems with perception cause youngsters to move too close or too far away, to trip or to stumble, to have difficulty manipulating objects: stacking, stringing, cutting, and drawing.

Youngsters who chew on pencils or bite may be responding to the need for *proprioception* sensory input, information from joint, muscle and tendon receptors. Proprioceptive input communicates to the brain when and how muscles are contracting or stretching, when and how joints are bending, extending, being pulled or compressed. Occupational therapists have found youngsters decrease biting when given surgical tubing or hard plastic drinking straws to chew on. Making a necklace out of the tubing with a knot in front provides a handy knot that can be chewed on whenever the youngsters feels like it.

Motivation

The lack of motivation and interest demonstrated by youngsters with FASD/FDE is in contrast to the inquisitiveness and fascination normally found in youngsters excited about learning. This lack of internal interest requires instruction that is heavily adult-directed. External motivation using rewards for effort in addition to success is required for youngsters who lack intrinsic motivation. Often ignored by youngsters who lack intrinsic motivation, routine and ritual help assure that basic grooming and hygiene is accomplished: brushing teeth, hair combing, bathing, and dressing. Perform these tasks using a schedule, at the same time, in the same location each day.

We expect children to be physically and mentally active, to spontaneously initiate, provoked by their natural curiosity and desire to make sense of the world; to use self-directed problem solving and experimentation. Youngsters with FASD/FDE may not initiate. They need play skills training before activities like free time with a variety of choices will be useful. Train children to make decisions for themselves by gradually expanding the choices available. Billie reports, that her grandson Jamal, will get up, dress himself and go outside, but then he would just stay in the yard at home unless prompted from others to play. His peers have accepted this and are the ones to initiate activities.

Incorporate sounds, sights, smells, and textures that motivate or interest students into learning situations. For instance, the youngster that favors sound can use recordings of stories to learn facts and language usage. Youngsters with FASD/FDE often have apparently meaningless preferences and attractions that motivate their behavior. Incorporating even a meaningless preference into the learning situation may increase the amount of time a student attends to a task. For example, I worked with a youngster, Eric, who was obsessed with maps and numbers. He took exceptional delight learning to read street names and applying simple math concepts to explaining directions on the maps he drew. Using an obsessive interest as a tool, he was learning: math, reading, writing, communication, and on-task follow through skills. Teachers that look for, build on, respond to, and encourage each child's interests and motivations will help their students develop a sense of competence that comes from acceptance, in addition to acquiring knowledge and skills.

Children understand and remember information that is within their developmental level, and are more likely to persist with tasks that involve their own physical, social, emotional, and intellectual experiences. Presenting material within a familiar cultural framework provides consistency and an inner-logic. Looking at the cultural patterns by which a student's family lives can suggest a variety of teaching methods. For example, some ethnic groups learn well when information is presented in a social conversational interchange. Other ethnic groups readily understand information that is presented with numerical facts. Other ethnic groups work well as part of a team. Provide opportunities to apply new learnings to situations that are meaningful, responsive to individual cultural differences, in addition to ability and interests. Children easily demonstrate their abilities through familiar cultural styles. Culture matters.

Reinforcement

Conditioning reinforcement techniques were the core of early behaviorists' learning theories. In Pavlovian conditioning, Pavlov's dog associated a stimulus with a previously unrelated response through the repeated presentation of a neutral stimulus. For example, a dog hears a bell (neutral stimulus) before being given food. Eventually, salivation (the conditioned response) is elicited by the sound of the bell alone (Gregory 1989). Give students feedback, specify what they are doing right. Positive reinforcers, which satisfy social needs increase learning acquisition. A primary function of positive reinforcement is to tell the child clearly what you want: "Thank you for putting the balls in the PE box." Specific verbal and nonverbal statements combined with praise clarify exactly what is expected, and to continually recognize the child's attempts.

Rewarding undesirable behavior with *attention reinforces* that behavior, increasing the likelihood it will continue, rather than decreasing how often it occurs. A common reinforcement error is giving a child's inappropriate comments and negative behavior attention, **ignore** undesirable and inappropriate behavior.

Attend to children who are behaving appropriately, just walking toward and standing beside students who are contributing positively encourages positive behavior in all students. There is a direct link between the student's response, the reinforcement, and the student's needs, physical or social. A thank you and a smile are powerful tools.

Decision-Making

Youngsters provided daily opportunities to make small decisions within a limited range of choices, learn to make and to take responsibility for choices. Joan Marguis, a social worker, offers choices within a set structure, "your three choices are." Robin Lindsley gives her kindergarten student's three choices. Chris Amos also limits choice options, her prekindergarten youngsters are given options which encourage them to exercise freedom of choice while developing decision-making skills. Children may need training and direction before they can make good choices and engage in productive free-time independent activities. I have personally watched in amazement and disbelief at the consistency with which some youngsters choose unsafe unconstructive inappropriate activities when exercising freedom of choice, who seem to have a proclivity against constructive behavior. The decision-making required for freedom of choice must be nourished and taught with the same attention given to learning other skills.

EVALUATION

The individual educational plan focus for each youngsters is to reach maximum potential within their fund of capabilities; based on present and future skills needed at home, in the school, and in the community.

Continuous evaluation detects subtle changes, providing the necessary information to design appropriate interventions. Does the youngster have a typical style of problem solving, of remembering, a modality preference? Adjust methods and materials to individual proficiencies within the student's learning style preferences. Ongoing observation and assessment of a child's responses to curriculum, lessons, and play activities are essential to planning curriculum and instruction. Documenting the length of time a student can focus on one task provides the information needed to structure assignments so that they can be completed in that length of time. Robin Lindsley has found that teachers have to reinvent curriculum and instructional strategies for each student because each "child is a different case." First, she analyzes a task, then breaks each task into small steps, then she presents instruction in this series of small steps. She presents the lesson, then reviews the lesson.

Evaluation of behavior during transition time provides an excellent opportunity to observe acting out, and to see examples of behaviors a youngster is having the most trouble with. Close observation of a child's behavior at transition times will reveal how the child uses skills, organizes and carries out a task, handles stress, copes with obstacles and reacts to change. Remain alert for chances to see a new skill used: responses, sensory preferences, and adaptations to new situations. Reactions to an unanticipated event, to an interruption, can be an opportunity for evaluation. Are perceptual preferences demonstrated: auditory, verbal, visual, tactile, kinesthetic?

Look for islands of competencies; what behavior is the child exhibiting? How are nonverbal behaviors used to communicate? How long can the child engage in an activity? What cognitive processes are involved? How does the child use skills during play, at transition times, and while engaged in self-help activities? How are behaviors used to establish communication? Does the child look at the speaker, at peers, or at the activity or object being referred to? How does the child use peers and adults to meet needs and solve problems? Answers to such questions lead to successfully adjusting an educational program to meet the student's developing and changing skills.

Formal testing in conjunction with daily evaluation helps determine the type of intervention needed and whether a child is likely to be able to lead an independent life as an adult. Medical and psychological evaluation can help determine the range of the child's learning disability, suggesting for example, whether or not medical management is needed along with skill development. A multidisciplinary team of specialists contribute expertise to devising appropriate remedial programs and exploring techniques with educators, speech therapists, physical therapists, occupational therapists, and other specialists' working with the youngster.

Testing is based on the hypothesis that abilities are correlated with later success. Two basic types of tests are norm-referenced and criterion-referenced. The purpose of *norm-referenced* testing is to determine a group or a student's grade level achievement compared with other students' of the same age, each student takes a complete test.

The purpose of a *criterion-referenced* test, is to determine the extent to which student objectives are being achieved, a percentage score is used to reflect the number of items correct for a specific objective. Each student is tested on items assigned to evaluate specific skills. Test results direct teaching to an individual child's performance. Many special needs students will be given tests that are criterion-referenced to determine specific competencies, and as a means to encourage learning.

Standardized comparisons inform professional judgment regarding the child's abilities and performance, as long as the assessments correlate with the skills that have been taught. Since the goal of assessment is to be able to develop a balanced program based on a student's abilities and individual characteristics, information on children with special needs should be as complete as possible. A comprehensive assessment needs to include information from formal standardized tests, behavioral observation, informal testing; in addition to interviews with the student and the parent.

There is no one formal assessment that is useful for the variety of skills exhibited in the special needs population, existing assessments must be used and adapted, modifications for test administration procedures can elicit data otherwise unavailable. *Test beyond the standardized criteria to identify skill fragments.*

Table 17. Testing Modifications.

Diagnostic evaluations and classroom subject assessment

Psychological Assessments:

- Allow the child to inspect the room and meet the examiner before the evaluation occurs. Sometimes including the child's teacher, tutor, or another familiar person will help.
- Determine in advance what reinforcement system has been effective.
- For the few children who are unable or unwilling to respond in the test situation, behavioral observation and structured interviews with educators, caretakers and parents can be sources of data.
- Adjusted readability level to the student.
- Narrow the scope of material to be tested.
- Oral instead of written tests
- Frequent short testing sessions.
- Give additional time to complete test
- Timed and untimed segments. Caution note: some skills, such as reading accuracy and fluency are most accurately assessed when timed.
- Use of projects to demonstrate proficiency in lieu of tests
- Conformation of findings in various settings is needed to determine validity for a specific child.
- Interpret results with caution recognizing that qualifying statements may be the most significant section of the evaluation.

General Assessments:

- Use visual cues to help child attend to and understand what you're saying.
- Get visual attention before giving directions.
- Repeat and simplify instructions
- Change to a different kind of task or a similar task at an easier level.
- Choose a test that reflects the various abilities of the child.
- Choose a test that measures concrete and abstract thinking skills.
- Due to language deficits, a student may need visually clear and self explanatory materials accompanied by gestures and direct physical guidance.
- Adapt language to child's level. Be concrete and specific, use short sentences and omit unnecessary words.
- Choose a test that provides separate measures of language and non-language skills.
- Allow student to give shorter answers to questions on a written assignment such as single word or phrase answers.
- Periodically check to see if students remember what they've learned in a previous lesson.

Adapted from: Mann, P. H., Suiter, P. A., & McClung, R M. (1992) and recommendations from school psychologists and teachers.

Chapter 9

EDUCATIONAL SERVICES

This chapter describes ways to fit the educational program to the child, with goals directed at acquiring essential skills and strategies that can be used for learning throughout life: maintaining behavioral, academic, self-care, and vocational gains, with ongoing support. Youngsters with neurological impairments and other disabilities provide a history of techniques and service directions for professionals working with children who have deficits affecting learning and behavior, resulting from prenatal drug/alcohol exposure. Practical hands-on examples are presented: how teachers have solved specific, learning, on-task, and behavior management problems.

Youngsters with FASD/FDE need techniques to help them adapt to the excitement and energy of school. Classroom experiences can include support services from a paraeducator aid, a speech and language specialist, an adaptive physical education teacher, a physical therapist, an occupational therapist, a school social worker, a school psychologist, and a school nurse.

Schools have established a multidisciplinary team model set up to provide the external support necessary to coordinate services for students with handicapping conditions requiring an Individualized Education Plan (IEP), and for students with comorbidities that require general medical and/or mental health services. Educational, parenting, and social support interventions are designed to modify the effects of prenatal drug/alcohol exposure; thus, allowing the youngster to develop full potential. It is often not the IQ or cognitive ability that is the source of a students problems, but the level of functional ability demanded. Case managers at school or family advocacy specialists can integrate this support for parents. Problems in adulthood, loss of employment or increased involvement with the criminal justice system can be ameliorated with adequate services.

Table 18. Top Ten Skills.

Academic Related Skills

 1. Able to stay on task (in the absence of teacher direction)
 2. Able to move from one activity to another cooperatively
 3. Able to complete academic work independently
 4. Able to sit at a desk and work independently without disturbing others
 5. Able to sit and attend to tasks in a group situation
 6 Tries to complete a task before giving up
 7. Demonstrates the basic academic skills sufficient to keep up with school curriculum
 8. Able to participate in large group activities
 9. Able to follow a variety of two and three-step directions
10. Able to use a variety of materials appropriately

Social Skills

 1. Initiates interactions with peers
 2. Participates with enthusiasm in work and play tasks
 3. Able to assist peers with some activity
 4. Displays an understanding of sharing
 5. Displays a good self-image
 6. Responds to name when called
 7. Displays an understanding of sharing
 8. Takes care of own toileting needs without assistance
 9. Responds to warning words
10. Social skills sufficient to allow for appropriate interactions with peers and teachers.

Reprinted with permission: Top ten skills educators report as critical to classroom success. Based on a literature search by Tim Lewis, Ph.D. University of Missouri 1995.

The classroom must change, the child can't. How can the room be modified to help the student? How can learning environments provide the nurturing, safety, and support youngsters need to learn new tasks.

change the behavior—change the environment

Robin Lindsley, a early childhood development specialist, like many other teachers is finding youngsters with FASD/FDE among the regular student population, students who can function pretty well but not as well as most others. Designed to fit the needs of students with a wide range of skills and problems, Robin's classroom provides a developmentally appropriate program that adjusts to the needs and developmental stages of individual students.

Students who do not learn spontaneously from a stimulating environment need creative learning environments that facilitate both independent and cooperative social development. The traditional classroom environment—with its noises, instructions, questions, interactions and distractions—can be too stimulating. Youngsters with FASD/FDE or similar disabilities, may be unable to adjust in even mildly stimulating environments: they don't like confusion, they don't find it creative. Children need to feel comfortable in a group, working individually, and in small groups. A challenge for the teacher is to structure the classroom environment in such a way that the dynamics of the group support the learning and social needs of all students. The group impact of youngsters on each other serves as a powerful tool for learning and social development. Whenever possible, utilize group resources rather than adult expertise.

Of particular importance is the **tolerance level of the teacher**. People differ in their willingness to put up with the noise and movement some children bring to class. Youngsters thrive in a comfortable secure environment where they feel the teacher is on their side and that they can get help in a predictable safe environment responsive to the variety of physical, intellectual, and emotional needs of all students.

CLASSROOM ENVIRONMENT

Children need a setting in which classroom materials and equipment can be removed to reduce stimuli, or added to enrich activities. Hands-on involvement in learning is facilitated by having small work areas devoted to specific skills, *activity centers*. Dividing a classroom up into work areas is especially useful for youngsters who have difficulty sitting at a desk, who need places for freedom of movement, and hands-on use of concrete materials: young children learn by manipulating their environment (Restak 1979). Learning by doing, experiential learning, may be needed by verbally fluent students with limited comprehension, or students who have problems actually doing what they can verbally describe. Activity centers used for early childhood education can be adapted for the older youngster with special needs. Robin Lindsley has found that youngsters with FASD/FDE frequently choose listening activity centers. They calm down when at the listening centers. Robin has children make a tape of their own voices, then use head phones for independent listening. Teachers find when students are doing something worthwhile at an activity-center, they are free to provide individual instruction to others.

Activity centers for older intermediate grade youngsters focus on listening, speaking, reading, and writing. The time for each activity ranges from thirty minutes to an hour, and it is best to limit the number of students at each center to less than five. Activity center subjects include: computer, listening, chalkboard/feltboard, writing, reading, math, art, and games. Students explore their interests, manipulate materials, and develop the skills needed to focus on one task at a time (Lindsley 1984). For example, a writing area could be supplied with materials used for writing, dictionaries, pencils, paper, and computers. A math area could have work sheets, counters, math games, manipulatives, and daily questions. Teachers have the freedom to give individual attention while other students remain interested and busy. Use of activity centers in the early grades provide opportunities for youngsters to acquire group work skills, and for cooperative learning in small groups with a focus on the teamwork necessary to complete projects and explore concepts. Successful groups have been taught *how* to work in a group (Black 1992).

CURRICULUM

Keeping in mind the goals of a curriculum, what can students with special needs do differently, what modifications can be made, so they can learn the skills others have? Two fundamental curriculum considerations are the characteristics of the learner, including capacity and state of prior knowledge, and the nature of the materials to be learned (pictures, stories, expository texts, maps). What tasks and skills are required of the learner; rote recall, recognizing inconsistencies, following instructions, comprehension? Flexible instructional routines along with appropriate curriculum materials support each student's growth. Ask, is there is a good match between the student's strengths and learning style, and with the curriculum material and instructional techniques used? Are opportunities for the student to answer, in a response style comfortable to the child, included and encouraged? Is instruction presented in a logical sequence? Are the goals of instruction and expectations for student performance clear and specific? After introducing new concepts or skills, is sufficient time allowed for practice, review, and elaboration before other new concepts or skills are introduced?

Table 19. Curriculum Instructional Materials Evaluation.

Learner Characteristics

- Is the material appropriate for the learner's interest, social and intellectual ability level?
- Does the student have the necessary intellectual, motor, and language competence?
- Does the material use student input and interests?
- Does the material require prerequisite learner skills?
- Is the material flexible, permitting self-pacing by the learner?
- Is the material chronologically age appropriate and grade level placement compatible?

Teachers Critique

- Does the material have appropriate sequential development?
- Does the material have different levels of abstraction and a range of language approaches to deal with concepts from simple concrete ideas to more complex thinking?
- Are the instructional activities related to real-life situations?
- Is the readability appropriate for the intended population: vocabulary, language structure and length of sentences (e. g., age and grade levels)?
- Supplementary materials: is the content comparable to regular class materials, varying in size, level of difficulty, or format?
- Is the material compatible with other materials and techniques being used?
- Does the material coordinate well with other subject areas?
- Are instructional technique modifications provided for varying types of teaching and learning styles?
- Is follow-up for previous lessons built into lesson plans, as well as pointing to follow-up for the current lesson?
- Is sufficient repetition, review, and reinforcement of skills, provided?
- Are activities aimed at helping students remember what they are learning?
- Are opportunities to rehearse or practice newly acquired information provided?

Adapted from the contributions of educators in my graduate courses, and Mann, P. H., Suiter, P. A., & McClung, R. M. (1992); Knight, D. & Wadsworth, D. (1993).

INCLUSION

Federal law mandates that educational services are to be provided in the least restrictive environment. The challenge of *inclusion*, joining specialized classrooms and services with the regular classroom, is the coordination of available services and staff to provide an optimal learning environment. Placement in a regular education classroom is not legally mandated by the "least restrictive environment" policy. School districts are required to offer a continuum of services for disabled children. The mandate is to provide the most *appropriate* education, with the goal to maximize a student's level of functioning within the limits of their disability, keeping a focus on the knowledge and skills necessary to function as independently as possible.

Placement decisions are strongly influenced by the perceptions of school administrators. A survey revealed principals were more likely to place students in less restrictive settings if they have had positive experiences with students who have disabilities, and if the principal has had exposure to special education concepts (Praisner 2003). Robin Lindsley has found teachers can't use inclusion without support. You can't just add youngsters to overloaded teachers. "If students fail, it really isn't the least restrictive environment." It's the school's responsibility to provide a learning atmosphere that includes opportunities for participation, promoting student responsibility and socialization.

"Imagine being dropped into a setting where people functioned at an intellectual level perhaps 50 or more IQ points above yours where their comments, jokes and conversations occurred on a level far above your capacity to comprehend, and where your infrequent inclusion into their activities and conversations was largely a function of their kindness and patience" (Rimland, B. 1990). Music class provides an excellent opportunity to increase youngsters tolerance of stimulation. Combining two and three classes for music can help students get ready to be included into traditional classrooms, sparking with energy.

A written Individualized Educational Plan (IEP) is required for all students receiving special education services. This IEP clarifies both objectives and specifies goal standards: exactly what the student and the educational service providers are expected to do.

Table 20. Individualized Education Plan (IEP).

The following information will likely be required as a teacher's contribution to an IEP, written in collaboration with a multidisciplinary team.

Content Area/Subject:

Instructor:

Present Skill Level:

Subject:

> Academic and Social Goals:
>
> Social/Physical Environment:
>
> > (adaptations and considerations):
>
> Level of Personal Assistance:
>
> Instructional Techniques:
>
> Curriculum Materials and Sequence:
>
> Classroom Management Procedures:
>
> Motivational Techniques:
>
> Evaluation - Standard of Performance Criteria:

Keep in Mind

- Your state or district may require additional information on the IEP.
- Communicate ideas so that other teachers and specialists as well as parents will understand the information.
- Home-school partnership: do the student's parents think the skills are important for both current and future needs?
- Inclusion tip: rethinking the traditional paradigm of schooling and the students day, may be needed to provide students with special needs the best learning experience.
- Consider joint enrollment with private schools specializing in services focusing on a specific disability, or half-day programs for students unable to tolerate a full-day.
- Adaptations are desirable given the challenges of class size, the range of student differences, and teacher planning time.
- Orient both student and classmates to unfamiliar equipment.
- Behavioral management techniques need to fit within classroom rules and the schoolwide discipline system (while not compromising the student with unrealistic expectations).
- Will personal one-to-one assistance be needed to ensure participation (volunteer, per, other)?

Student

- For many children normal development cannot be the goal. Rather, the goal is to improve their adaptation within the limits of their disability.
- Goals and objectives: does the student have the necessary intellectual, physical, behavioral, and language competence to attain the learning objectives.
- To keep the student challenged, take into consideration the students attitudes and interests.
- Is the functionality of goals and the instructional content appropriate for meeting the student's personal-social, daily living, and occupational adjustment needs?

- Determine functionality of goals with a specific focus on the knowledge and skills necessary to function as independently as possible in the home, school, and community.
- Specify how goals will be demonstrated—students response requirements.

CLASSROOM MANAGEMENT OF BEHAVIOR

Behavioral management goals and techniques need to fit both within classroom rules and the school-wide discipline system, while not compromising the student with unrealistic expectations. First ask, does the student have the necessary intellectual, physical, behavioral, and language competence to attain the behavioral objectives. Inconsistent responses complicate the situation, children who show different responses to the same events on different days, may be neurologically damaged in the areas of the brain that deal with behavior. For example, the great majority of the time Jack hangs up his coat on his specific hanger; even if peers push and shove, or hang their coat on his hanger. Then one day he just keeps his coat on, refusing to hang it up, and pushes a classmate. When responding to a child's misbehavior, try to identify what the child seems to want before dealing with the misbehavior. Behavior that absolutely looks like it originates from the meanest motivation may not be, and can most successfully be dealt with using a caring nonjudgmental calm demeanor, recognizing that every misbehavior does not warrant attention.

Youngsters with FASD/FDE can have behaviors that demand creative learning environments, and teachers that maintain an accepting perspective about misbehavior. Beth Caruso, a prekindergarten teacher, has extensive experience working with handicapped youngsters: deaf, blind, language delayed, and developmentally delayed. In her prekindergarten classroom the class has accepted continuing their activities in spite of a youngster who cannot stop and redirect disruptive behavior, she finds "the challenge is maintaining the rest of the classroom." This youngster can't stop fighting, or talking, or screaming, "once they get on a track, they just can't get off the track." Beth and her students continue with the class activities, "we just sing over him when he can't stop screaming."

Teachers have found a universal cue to "stop" a behavior, which can be used as a signal to stop for any behavior, an effective external management tool. For example, the teacher shows the student a purple X as a symbol to stop. Once learned, this concrete consistent signal to stop can be used in all situations, helping the student understand what to do.

Youngsters who are easily frustrated and irritable may need time-out to reduce overstimulation and gain control when integrating into the traditional classroom, filled with the vitality of youngsters who are able to settle themselves down. Voluntary and involuntary time-out with the use of study-carrels (three-sided partitions placed on a child's desk to enclose their work area), block out classroom distractions, and keep students on task. Teachers find most students request and use study-carrels and time-out when they need to reduce the classroom stimulation and organize themselves. Students respond well to small spaces and welcome the small enclosed areas that study-carrels provide. Robin Lindsey, offers the use of a study-carrel as free choice for all students, opening up the opportunity to advise overstimulated students to use them, "You may need to use the study-carrel now." Students' can choose to adjust their environment within a distracting classroom. Beth, as many other teachers have been forced to do, found a practical functional technique for reducing stimulation and helping define boundaries, for the one drug effected youngster in her prekindergarten. Beth helps this youngster "define her space," as she puts her arms around the youngster and says "this is your space." Like the use of desks with older students or the carpet squares during circle in kindergarten classrooms, Beth provides a specific concrete definition of space. She can put her arms around the student and say "this is your space" during any activity. Time-out and use of study-carrels help reduce, and help manage the flood of sensory information found in the classroom.

HOME-SCHOOL PARTNERSHIP

Teachers need the support of parents: partners in the educational process. Keep in mind, parents may have learning disabilities themselves, and/or find it difficult to focus when discussing their child with educators. Use of instructional strategies with parents can improve communication effectiveness such as, repetition, and modeling using verbal explanations with nonverbal actions. A genuine interest in the child's and the parent's well-being facilitate this home-school partnership. Home visits can be made to identify what skills the child needs, parental concerns, and what the family needs are. Based on what is available in the child's home, design activities that fit both the classroom and the home environment. Ask parents, do they think the skills taught are important for both their child's current and future needs? Encourage parents to ask questions. Beth recommends that educators "put the investment in the family." She lets the child and family know she, the teacher is on their side. She has parents come and work with their children in class, so that both home and school use the same strategies, integrating classroom learning into their daily habits at home. Involve parents in information gathering, identifying problems, problem solving, and teaching. Incorporating the family integrates the child's environment, providing reciprocal home-school-community learning opportunities.

Table 21. Home Visit Questions.

How Did/Does the Child

- Appear alert?
- Try new tasks?
- Show signs of empathy?
- Show appropriate emotions?
- What communication techniques are used?
- How does the child get needs met?
- Does the child's language differ from normal? How?
- How are the child's unique differences reflected in the child's learning?
- What changes would the parent like to see?

How does the Parent

- Initiate positive interactions and affection with the child?
- Enjoy reciprocal interactions with the child?
- Respond to the child's affection?
- Respond to the child's overtures?
- Understand the child's communication?
- Respond to the child's expressions of positive and negative feelings?
- Respond with reasonable expectations?

In addition to home visits, Beth facilitates home-school communication using informal notes. A notebook or e-mail sent back and forth between parents and teachers to discuss events at home and school;

thus, integrating and organizing the youngsters experiences. This additional focus on daily routines and special events increases external organization for poorly organized youngsters. Helping parents understand their child's strengths and weaknesses facilitates the goal of making the home environment supportive of emotional and cognitive development.

Parent/Caregiver Support

The emotional bond between parent and child is strengthened by interaction and involvement. Nevertheless, parents often find children with FASD/FDE hard to understand, hard to like, and difficult to live with. For example, would you understand a deaf child's behavior if you didn't know the child was deaf? A review of studies on parental care noted that child behavior affected adult caregiving (Hans 2002). Understanding that behavior is more likely due to neurological problems than to a rejection of the adults attentions, or values, can stop potentially dysfunctional parent-infant interactions before detrimental patterns become established. It's important for each child's emotional development to feel that adults like them and value their company.

Results of a medical diagnosis, IQ testing, and a teacher evaluation help parents set realistic expectations for their child's behavior and performance level. Unrealistic expectations for children may exacerbate dysfunctional parent-child interactions, and have been correlated with a potential for child abuse (Sachs and Hall 1991). The normal-looking youngster with a prodigious verbal repertoire devoid of substance is a violation of our expectations. Hence, identification of a deficit allows the child, the parents, and the teachers to better understand: to look first at biology rather than poor intent.

Beth's focus is to help parents understand it's not the child's fault. Once parents understand the influence of neurobehavior deficits on the child's behavior, they feel better about their efforts and the child's progress. Beth feels her respect for parents has contributed to successful family involvement. When making "child-centered" home visits, she focuses on the child's abilities, repeatedly stating, "Look at what he can do." Have parents encourage the child to engage in activities that provide opportunities to feel competent. She persuades parents to notice and respond positively to good behavior. Positive interactions between parent and child are strengthened by instruction and problem-solving strategies that fit the child and bypass deficient skill areas. Beth has found "home visits are an investment in teacher time that pays off," improving the quality of learning and behavior control in the classroom. Facilitation of a home-school partnership is a fundamental part of the youngster's educational program.

> We all want our parents to accept who we are, warts—deficits—talents—and all.

ACCESSING EDUCATIONAL SERVICES

School services available to youngsters reflect the values, priorities, and assets of a community. Billie, a health coordinator for Head Start nurses, has taken care of her fifteen-year-old grandson since birth. Despite the possible advantage she may have over other parents due to her professional experience within the school system, she has nevertheless had problems. Billie describes her experience with the school system in securing services for Jamal as a "fight all the way through." Jamal, who has difficulty dealing with change of any kind, was often moved to different classrooms. While the school district was looking for the best educational fit for Jamal, he was placed in some inappropriate classrooms. She found that students receiving special education services change programs and classrooms often, losing valuable learning time adjusting to new situations. Billie's grandson's limited abstract reasoning and social judgment resulted in his imitating the behaviors of other students. When placed in classrooms designed for emotionally disturbed children, he imitated their negative behaviors. When integrated into classrooms for regular youngsters, he imitated normal behaviors.

Medical foster moms' say they need instruction on "how to deal with the school," to get the schools to recognize that these children are disabled, not bad or uncooperative. They describe long meetings with school special education departments, trying to get services for youngsters with mild FASD/FDE. Youngsters who do not meet the state's guidelines for a handicapping condition, are not eligible for services. The student people describe as "falling through the cracks," has difficulty learning in a traditional classroom, but doesn't fit the criteria necessary for services, may be the student that would profit from services and interventions not commonly used in traditional classrooms. Actually, this is the very child who might be the most helped by services, because this is the least damaged and most remediable of the students' with handicaps. Absolutely the best advice to parents was presented by a speaker at a parent training group. First, she advised, accept that all teachers will not have the background necessary to educate a child with the particular disability their child has. Second, write up a concise description of their child's disability noting the instructional strategies that have been successful, keep this description to less than three pages, make copies, and each year give this information to all new teachers. One more of the valuable tools needed to help youngsters get an education, and to graduate from school with work and life skills.

Appendix

WHAT IS FAS?

It is said that we cannot understand another man's problems unless we walk in his shoes. So let's do just that. Let's imagine. . . .

It is Tuesday of the first week of school and you are on your way to your second day of kindergarten. You are a lot shorter than most of your class-mates and skinnier, too. Now that you are five you are aware of this. You also are aware—in fact, you have been told—that you have this "thing" that makes you small. It's called fetal alcohol syndrome and it has something to do with your mother drinking alcohol before you were born, but you really don't understand that. There are a lot of things you don't understand, like what to do first when you are told to do lots of things at once. Then you get scared and mixed up, but instead of asking for help you might push the person next to you. You wouldn't know why you pushed him, but it seems to be some-thing you just have to do!

Something else you don't understand is how to walk in a line. You keep bumping into the kids in front of you and touching things—like the ribbons at the end of Suzie's braids. The ribbons were shiny and pretty. You just had to feel them! So then you got into trouble and it was horrible.

After you said you were sorry in front of everybody, and the whole line stood still watching, and then the whole line started walking again, you got into trouble again! You kicked the boy behind you! Right in the shin and did he scream. Well, you couldn't help it! You felt like you were being squished, like a pickle on a McDonald's hamburger—squished and pulled apart. You hate to be touched sometimes and people in this school keep bumping into you and touching you. What else could you DO but kick to get people out of the way.

And here you are back at school again today. Finally, you go on down the hall wishing all the noise would go away. Kids are talking, teachers are talking, a loudspeaker is calling something about a phone call and you are confused. You clutch your mother's hand, but then you get really mad at her.

Why can't she make it all better? It's all her fault! She pushes you gently into the room and smiles good-by.

You walk into the room. It's a great room! Every wall is covered with bright colored pictures and things are hanging from the ceiling; things like A B C letters and whales and fish. They're moving in the air at the end of wool strings. You want to touch and see everything all at once. You love the dove in her cage, and the sound she makes, too. Everything is great here! You love the piano and want to play it right now! But there's the fish to look at, and the hamster, and the sand table, and the books, and the dress-up clothes, and the containers with all those big colored blocks and stuff. But . . . you also want to get away because your heart is starting to beat fast and you feel like you do in the back of a moving car–a little sick. Maybe you can crawl under the table and hide. You start doing that but then something happens. You see a truck and you pick it up and you throw it! It hits Billy in the head and you get so scared and mad that you push the girl next to you and she slams into the edge of the table. They start crying and you REALLY want to go home.

This is FAS.

(Reprinted with permission: Gloria Stuart, 2005)

REFERENCES

Aaron, P. G. (1981). Diagnosis and remediation of learning disabilities in children–
A neuropsychological key approach. In G. W. Hynd & J. E. Obrzt (Eds.).
Neuropsychological assessment and the school-age child (pp. 303–333). New York, NY:
Grune & Stratton.

Abel, E. L. (1984). *Fetal alcohol syndrome and fetal alcohol effects.* New York, NY:
Plenum Press.

Acker, D., Sachs, B. P., Tracey, K. J., Wise, W. E. (1983). Abruptio placentae associated with cocaine use. *American Journal of Obstetrics and Gynecology, 146* (2),
220–221.

Alkon, D. L. (1989, July). Memory storage and neural systems. *Scientific American,
261* (1), 42–50.

Annand, J. (2002). *More than accommodation: Overcoming barriers to effective treatment of
persons with both cognitive disabilities and chemical dependency.* Oregon: Nightwind.

Archibald, S. L., Fennema-Notestine, C., Gamst, A., Riley, E. P., Mattson, S. N., &
Jernigan, T. L. (2001). Brain dysmorphology in individuals with severe prenatal
alcohol exposure. *Developmental Medicine and Child Neurology, 43* (3), 148–154.

Arendt, R. E., Short, E. J., Singer, L. T., Minnes, S., Hewitt, J., Flynn, S., Carlson, L.,
Min, M. O., Klein, N., & Flannery, D. (2004). Children prenatally exposed to
cocaine: Developmental outcomes and environmental risks at seven years of
age. *Journal of Developmental and Behavioral Pediatrics, 25* (2), 83–90.

Arwood, E. L. (1983). *Pragmaticism: Theory and application.* Rockville, MD: Aspen
Systems.

Aslin, R. N. (1984). Sensory and perceptual constraints on memory in human
infants. In R. Kail & E. Spear (Eds.). *Comparative perspectives on the development of
memory* (pp. 39–64). Hillsdales, NJ: Lawrence Erlbaum Associates.

Astley, S. J., Clarren, S. K., Little, R. E., Sampson, P. D., Daling, J. R. (1992).
Analysis of facial shape in children gestationally exposed to marijuana, alcohol,
and/or cocaine. *Pediatrics, 89* (1), 67–77.

Astley, S. J., & Clarren, S. K. (1999). *Diagnostic guide for fetal alcohol syndrome and related conditions: The 4-digit diagnostic code, 2nd edition.* Seattle: University of
Washington.

Astley, S. J., Stachowiak, J., Clarren, S. K., & Clausen, C. (2002). Application of the
fetal alcohol syndrome facial photographic screening tool in a foster care population. *The Journal of Pediatrics, 141* (5), 712–717.

153

Autti-Ramo, I. (2002). Foetal alcohol syndrome–A multifaceted condition. *Developmental Medicine and Child Neurology, 44* (2), 141–144.

Autti-Ramo, I., Korkman, M., Hilakivi-Clarke, L., Lehtonen, M., Halmesmaki, E., Granstrom, M. L. (1992). Mental development of 2-year-old children exposed to alcohol in utero. *The Journal of Pediatrics, 120* (5), 740–746.

Bada, H. S., Bauer, C. R., Shankaran, S., Lester, B., Wright, L. L., Das, A., Poole, K., Smeriglio, V. L., Finnegan, L. P., & Maza, P. L. (2002). Central and autonomic system signs with in utero drug exposure. *Archives of Disease in Childhood, 87* (2), 106–112.

Baddeley, A. (1992). Working memory. *Science, 255* (5044), 556–559.

Baddeley A. D. (1976). *The psychology of memory.* New York, NY: Basic Books.

Baddeley, A. (1982). *Your memory: A user's guide.* New York, NY: Macmillan.

Baer, J. S., Sampson, P. D., Barr, H. M, Connor, P. D., & Streissguth, A. P. (2003). A 21-year longitudinal analysis of the effects of prenatal alcohol exposure on young adult drinking. *Archives General Psychiatry, 60* (4), 377–385.

Bandstra, E. S., Morrow, C. E., Vogel, A. L., Fifer, R. C., Ofir, A. Y., Dausa, A. T., Xue, L., & Anthony, J. C. (2002). Longitudinal influence of prenatal cocaine exposure on child language functioning. *Neurotoxicology and Teratology, 24* (3), 297–308.

Barr, H. M, & Streissguth, A. P. (2001). Identifying maternal self-reported alcohol use associated with fetal alcohol spectrum disorders. *Alcoholism Clinical and Experimental Research, 25* (2), 283–287.

Baumbach, J. (2002). Some implications of prenatal alcohol exposure for the treatment of adolescents with sexual offending behaviors. *Sexual Abuse: A Journal of Research and Treatment, 14* (4), 313–327.

Beaconsfield, P., Birdwood, G., Beaconsfield, R. (1980, August). The placenta. *Scientific American, 243* (2), 94–102.

Bhatara, V. S., Lovrein, F., Kirkeby, J., Swayze, V., Unruh, E., & Johnson, V. (2002). Brain function in fetal alcohol syndrome assessed by single photon emission computed tomography. *South Dakota Journal of Medicine, 55* (2), 59–62.

Black, S. (1992). Group learning. *The Executive Educator, 14* (9), 18–20.

Bloom, F. E., & Lazerson A. (1988). *Brain, mind, and behavior.* New York, NY: W. H. Freeman.

Bookstein, F. L., Streissguth, A. P., Sampson, P. D., Connor, P. D., & Barr, H. M. (2002). Corpus callosum shape and neuropsychological deficits in adult males with heavy fetal alcohol exposure. *NeuroImage, 15* (1), 233–251.

Bower, T. G. R. (1976, November). Repetitive processes in child development. *Scientific American, 235* (5), 38–47.

Bozarth, M. A., & Wise, R. A. (1985). Toxicity associated with long-term intravenous heroin and cocaine self-administration in the rat. *Journal of the American Medical Association, 254* (1), 81–83.

Brazelton, T. B., & Cramer, B. G. (1991). *The earliest relationship.* New York, NY: Addison-Wesley.

Brown, J. V., Bakeman, R., Coles, C. D., Platzman, K. A., & Lynch, M. E. (2004). Prenatal cocaine exposure: A comparison of 2-year-old children in parental and nonparental care. *Child Development, 75* (4), 1282–1295.

Burkett, G., Yasin, S., & Palow, D. (1990). Perinatal implications of cocaine exposure. *Journal of Reproductive Medicine, 35* (1), 35–42.

Burd, L, Cotsonas-Hassler, T. M., Martsolf, J. T., & Kerbeshian, J. (2003). Recognition and management of fetal alcohol syndrome. *Neurotoxicology and Teratology, 25* (6), 681–688.

Burd, L., Klug, M. G., Martsolf, J. T., & Kerbeshian, J. (2003). Fetal alcohol syndrome: neuropsychiatric phenomics. *Neurotoxicology and Teratology, 25* (6), 697–705.

Calder, A. J., Lawrence, A. D., & Young, A. W. (2001). Neuropsychology of fear and loathing. *National Review of Neuroscience, 2,* 352–363.

Carney, L. J., & Chermak, G. D. (1991). Performance of American Indian children with fetal alcohol syndrome on the test of language development. *Journal of Communication Disorders, 24* (2), 123–134.

Carpenter, P. A., Just, M. A., & Reichle, E. D. (2000). Working memory and executive function: Evidence from neuroimaging. *Current Opinion in Neurobiology, 10,* 195–199.

Chambers, C. D., & Jones, K. L. (2002). Is genotype important in predicting the fetal alcohol syndrome? [editorials]. *The Journal of Pediatrics, 141* (6), 751–752.

Chasnoff, I. J., Anson, A., Hatcher, R., Stenson, H., Iaukea, K., & Randolph, L. (1998). Prenatal exposure to cocaine and other drugs: outcome at four to six years. *Annals of the New York Academy of Sciences, 846,* 314–328.

Chasnoff, I. J., Griffith, D. R., Freier, C., Murray, J. (1992). Cocaine/polydrug use in pregnancy: Two-year follow-up. *Pediatrics, 89* (2), 284–289.

Chasnoff, I. J. (1991b). Cocaine and pregnancy: clinical and methodologic issues. *Clinics in Perinatology, 18* (1), 113–123.

Chasnoff, I. J., & Griffith, D. R. (1989). Cocaine: Clinical studies of pregnancy and the newborn. *Annals of the New York Academy of Sciences, 562,* 260–266.

Chasnoff, I. J. (1989). Cocaine, pregnancy, and the neonate. *Women and Health, 15* (3), 23–35.

Chasnoff, I. J. (1987, May). Perinatal effects of cocaine. *Contemporary OB/GYN, 29* (5), 163–179.

Chasnoff, I. J., Burns, K. A., Burns, W. J., & Schnoll, S. H. (1986). Prenatal drug exposure: Effects on neonatal and infant growth and development. *Neurobehavioral Toxicology and Teratology, 8* (4), 357–362.

Chasnoff, I. J., Burns, W. M., Schnoll, S. H., & Burns, K. A. (1985). Cocaine use in pregnancy. *New England Journal of Medicine, 313* (11), 666–669.

Chasnoff, I. J., Hatcher, R., & Burns, W. (1982). Polydrug- and methadone-addicted newborns: A continuum of impairment? *Pediatrics, 70* (2), 210–213.

Chavez, G. F., Cordero, J. F., & Becerra, J. E. (1989). Leading major congenital malformations among minority groups in the United States, 1981–1986. *Journal of the American Medical Association, 261* (2), 205–209.

Chomsky, N. (1986). *Knowledge of language: It's nature, origin, and use.* Westport, CT: Greenwood Press.

Clarren, S. (2005). Dr Sterling Clarren's keynote address to the Yukon 2002 Prairie Northern Conference on Fetal Alcohol Syndrome. *http://come-over.to/ FAS/Whitehorse/WhitehorseArticleSC1.htm.* Accessed [06/2005].

Clarren, S. K., Olson, H. C., Clarren, S. G. B., & Astley, S. (2000). A child with fetal alcohol syndrome. In M. J. Guralnick (Ed.), *Interdisciplinary clinical assessment of young children with developmental disabilities* (pp. 307–326). Baltimore: Paul H. Brookes.

Cline, F. W. (1979). *Understanding and treating the severely disturbed child.* Evergreen, CO: Evergreen Consultants in Human Behavior.

Cloninger, C. R., Sigvardsson, S., & Bohman, M. (1996). Type I and Type II alcoholism: An update. *Alcohol Health and Research World, 20* (1), 18–23.

Connor, P. D., Sampson, P. D., Bookstein, F. L., Barr, H. M., & Streissguth, A. P. (2000). Direct and indirect effects of prenatal alcohol damage on executive function. *Developmental Neuropsychology, 18* (3), 331–354.

Connor, P. D., Streissguth, A. P., Sampson, P. D., Bookstein, F. L., & Barr, H. M. (1999). Individual differences in auditory and visual attention among fetal alcohol-affected adults. *Alcoholism: Clinical and Experimental Research, 23* (8), 1395–1402.

Corwin, M. J., Lester, B. M., Sepkoski, C., McLaughlin, S., Kayne, H., & Golub, H. L. (1992). Effects of in utero cocaine exposure on newborn acoustical cry characteristics. *Pediatrics, 89* (6), 1199–1203.

Covington, C. Y., Nordstrom-Klee, B., Ager, J., Sokol, R., & Delaney-Black, V. (2002). Birth to age 7 growth of children prenatally exposed to drugs: A prospective cohort study. *Neurotoxicology and Teratology, 24* (4), 489–496.

Crain, W. (1980). *Theories of development: Concepts and applications.* Englewood Cliffs, NJ: Prentice Hall.

Crick, F., & Koch, C. (2003). A framework for consciousness [commentary]. *Nature Neuroscience, 6* (2), 119–126.

Day, N. L., Leech, S. L., Richardson, G. A., Cornelius, M. C., Robles, N, & Larkby, C. (2002). Prenatal alcohol exposure predicts continued deficits in offspring size at 14 years of age. *Alcoholism Clinical and Experimental Research, 26* (10), 1584–1591.

Delaney-Black, V., Covington, C., Templin, T., Kershaw, T., Nordstrom-Klee, B., Ager, J., Clark, N., Surendran, S. M., & Sokol, R. J. (2000). Expressive language development of children exposed to cocaine prenatally: Literature review and report of a prospective cohort study. *Journal of Communication Disorders, 33* (6), 463–481.

Dolan, R. M., & Vuilleumier, P. (2003). Amygdala automaticity in emotional processing. *Annals of the New York Academy of Sciences, 985,* 348–355.

Dorris, M. (1989). *The broken cord.* New York, NY: Harper & Row.

Dow-Edwards, D. L., Freed, L. A., & Fico, T. A. (1990). Structural and functional effects of prenatal cocaine exposure in adult rat brain. *Developmental Brain Research, 57* (2), 263–268.

Ebbinghaus, H. (1964). *Memory a contribution to experimental psychology.* New York, NY: Dover.

Edwards, B. (1979). *Drawing on the right side of the brain.* Los Angeles, CA: J. P. Tarcher.

Eich, E. (1984). Memory for unattended events: Remembering with and without awareness. *Memory and Cognition, 12* (2), 105–111.

Eisen, L. N., Field, T. M., Bandstra, E. S., Roberts, J. P., Morrow, C., Larson, S. K., & Steele, B. M. (1991). Perinatal cocaine effects on neonatal stress behavior and performance on the Brazelton Scale. *Pediatrics, 88* (3), 477–480.

Eriksson, C. J., Fukunaga, T., Sarkola, T., Chen, W. J., Chen, C. C., Ju, J. M., Cheng, A. T., Yamamoto, H., Kohlenberg-Muller, K., Kimura, M., & Murayama, M. (2001). Functional relevance of human ADH polymorphism [symposium]. *Alcoholism Clinical and Experimental Research, 25* (5), 1575–1635.

Ernhart, C. B., Sokol, R. J., Martier, S., Moron, P., Nadler, D., Ager, J. W., & Wolf, A. (1987). Alcohol teratogenicity in the human: A detailed assessment of specificity, critical period, and threshold. *American Journal of Obstetrics and Gynecology, 156* (1), 33–39.

Eslinger, P. J. (1996). Conceptualizing, describing, and measuring components of executive function: A summary. In G. R. Lyon & N. A. Krasnegor (Eds.), *Attention, memory, and executive function* (pp. 367–395). Baltimore: Brookes.

Estenson, P. (2003, June). The value of psychotherapy for adults with fetal alcohol spectrum disorders. *Iceberg*, pp. 6–7.

Eyler, F. D., Behnke, M., Garvan, C. W., Woods, N. S. Wobie, K., & Conlon, M. (2001). Newborn evaluations of toxicity and withdrawal related to prenatal cocaine exposure. *Neurotoxicology and Teratology, 23* (5), 399–411.

Fahlberg, V. I. (1991). *A child's journey through placement*. Indianapolis, IN: Perspectives Press.

Famy, C., Streissguth, A. P., & Unis, A. S. (1998). Mental illness in adults with fetal alcohol syndrome or fetal alcohol effects. *The American Journal of Psychiatry, 155* (4), 552–554.

Ferretti, R. P. (1989). Problem solving and strategy production in mentally retarded persons. *Research in Developmental Disabilities, 10,* 19–31.

Fetters, L., & Tronick, E. Z. (1996). Neuromotor development of cocaine-exposed and control infants from birth through 15 months: Poor and poorer performance. *Pediatrics, 98* (5), 938–943.

Fields, R. D. (2004). The other half of the brain. *Scientific American, 290* (4), 54–61.

Forgas, J. P., Burnham, D. K., & Trimboli, C. (1988). Mood, memory, and social judgments in children. *Journal of Personality and Social Psychology, 54* (4), 697–703.

Frank, D. A., Augustyn, M., Knight, W. G., Pell, T., & Zuckerman, B. (2001). Growth, development, and behavior in early childhood following prenatal cocaine exposure: A systematic review. *The Journal of the American Medical Association, 285* (12), 1613–1625.

Frank, D. A., Jacobs, R. R., Beeghly, M., Augustyn, M., Bellinger, D., Cabral, H., & Heeren, T. (2002). Level of prenatal cocaine exposure and scores on the Bayley scales of infant development: Modifying effects of caregiver, early intervention, and birth weight. *Pediatrics, 110* (6), 1143–1152.

Gawin, F. H. (1991). Cocaine addiction: psychology and neurophysiology. *Science, 251,* 1580–1586.

Gendle, M. H., Strawderman, M. S., Mactutus, C. F., Booze, R. M., Levitsky, D. A., & Strupp, B. J. (2004). Prenatal cocaine exposure does not alter working memory in adult rats. *Neurotoxicology and Teratology, 26* (2), 319–329.

Giancola, P. R., & Mezzich, A. C. (2003). Executive functioning, temperament, and drug use involvement in adolescent females with a substance use disorder. *Journal of Child Psychology and Psychiatry, 44* (6), 857–866.

Giancola, P. R., Shoal, G. D., & Mezzich, A. C. (2001). Constructive thinking, executive functioning, antisocial behavior, and drug use involvement in adolescent females with a substance use disorder. *Experimental and Clinical Psychopharmacology, 9* (2), 215–227.

Gingras, J. L., O'Donnell, K. J., & Hume, R. F. (1990). Maternal cocaine addiction and fetal behavioral state. I: A human model for the study of sudden infant death syndrome. *Medical Hypotheses, 33* (4), 227–230.

Gingras, J. L., Weese-Mayer, D. E., Hume, R. F., & O'Donnell, K. J. (1992). Cocaine and development: Mechanisms of fetal toxicity and neonatal consequences of prenatal cocaine exposure. *Early Human Development, 31* (1), 1–24.

Gleason, M., Carnine, D., & Vala, N. (1991, February). Cumulative versus rapid introduction of new information. *Exceptional Children,* 353–358.

Golden, C. J. (1981). The Luria-Nebraska children's battery: Theory and formulation. In G. W. Hynd & J. E. Obrzt (Eds.). *Neuropsychological assessment and the school-age child* (pp. 277–302). New York, NY: Grune & Stratton.

Goldman-Rakic, P. S. (1992, September). Working memory and the mind. *Scientific American, 267* (3), 110–117.

Gopnik, A., Meltzoff, A. N., & Kuhl, P. K. (1999). *The scientist in the crib: What early learning tells us about the mind.* New York: HarperCollins.

Gregory, R. L. (Ed.). (1989). *The Oxford Companion to The Mind.* New York, NY: Oxford University Press.

Guerri, C., Pascual, M., & Renau-Piqueras, J. (2001). Glia and fetal alcohol syndrome. *Neurotoxicology, 22* (5), 593–599.

Hamann, S. (2003). Nosing in on the emotional brain. *Nature Neuroscience, 6* (2), 106–108.

Handler, A., Kistin, N., Davis, F., & Ferre, C. (1991). Cocaine use during pregnancy: Perinatal outcomes. *American Journal of Epidemiology, 133* (8), 818–825.

Hanley, W. B. (2002). Microcephaly and fetal alcohol syndrome [letters]. *The Journal of Pediatrics, 141* (3), 449.

Hans, S. L. (2002). Studies of prenatal exposure to drugs: Focusing on parental care of children. *Neurotoxicology and Teratology, 24* (3), 329–337.

He, N., Bai, J., Champoux, M., Suomi, S. J., & Lidow, M. S. (2004). Neurobehavioral deficits in neonatal rhesus monkeys exposed to cocaine in utero. *Neurotoxicology and Teratology, 26* (1), 13–21.

Hebb, D. O. (1949). *The Organization of Behavior.* New York: Wiley.

Heilman, K. M. (1978). Language and the brain: Relationship of localization of language function to the acquisition and loss of various aspects of language. In J. S. Chall & A. F. Mirsky (Eds.). *Education and the brain: The seventy seventh yearbook of the national society for the study of education part II* (pp. 143–168). Chicago, IL: The National Society for the Study of Education.

Hoyme, H. E., Jones, K. L., Dixon, S. D., Jewett, T., Hanson, J. W., Robinson, L. K., Msall, M. E., & Allanson, J. E. (1990). Prenatal cocaine exposure and fetal vascular disruption. *Pediatrics 85* (5), 743–747.

Hunt, M. (1982). *The universe within: A new science explores the human mind*. New York, NY: Simon and Schuster.

Hynd, G. W., Semrud-Clikeman, M., Lorys, A. R., Novey, E. S., Eliopulos, D., & Lyytinen, H. (1991). Corpus callosum morphology in attention deficit-hyperactivity disorder: Morphometric analysis of MRI. *Journal of Learning Disabilities, 24* (3), 141–146.

Johanson, C., & Fischman, M. W. (1989). The pharmacology of cocaine related to its abuse. *Pharmacological Reviews, 41* (1), 3–52.

Jones, K. L. (2003). From recognition to responsibility: Josef Warkany, David Smith, and the fetal alcohol syndrome in the 21st century. *Birth Defects Research (Part A) Clinical and Molecular Teratology, 67* (1), 13–20.

Jones, K. L. (1991). Developmental pathogenesis of defects associated with prenatal cocaine exposure: Fetal vascular disruption. *Chemical Dependency and Pregnancy, 18* (1), 139–146.

Jones, K. L., & Smith, D. W. (1973). Recognition of the fetal alcohol syndrome in early infancy. *The Lancet, 2* (7836), 999–1001.

Jones, K. L., Smith, D. W., Ulleland, C. N., & Streissguth, A. P. (1973). Pattern of malformation in offspring of chronic alcoholic mothers. *The Lancet, 1*, 1267–1271.

Jones, N. A., Field, T., Davalos, M., & Hart, S. (2004). Greater right frontal EEG asymmetry and nonemphathic behavior are observed in children prenatally exposed to cocaine. *International Journal of Neuroscience, 114*, 459–480.

Kaemingk, K. L., Mulvaney, S., & Halverson, P. T. (2003). Learning following prenatal alcohol exposure: Performance on verbal and visual multitrial tasks. *Archives of Clinical Neuropsychology, 18* (1), 33–47.

Kagan, J. (1972, March). Do infants think? *Scientific American, 226* (3), 74–82.

Kane, M. (1984). Cognitive styles of thinking and learning part one. *Academic Therapy, 19* (5), 527–536.

Kataria, S., Hall, C. W., Wong, M. M., & Keys, G. F. (1992). Learning styles of LD and NLD ADHD children. *Journal of Clinical Psychology, 48* (3), 371–378.

Kelly, S. J., Day, N., & Streissguth, A. P. (2000). Effects of prenatal alcohol exposure on social behavior in humans and other species. *Neurotoxicology and Teratology, 22* (2), 143–149.

Kerns, K. A., Don, A., Mateer, C. A., & Streissguth, A. P. (1997). Cognitive deficits in nonretarded adults with fetal alcohol syndrome. *Journal of Learning Disabilities, 30* (6), 685–693.

Kessler, R. C., Nelson, C. B., McGonagle, K. A., Edlund, M. J., Frank, K. G., & Leaf, P. J. (1996). The epidemiology of co-occurring mental disorders and substance use disorders in the national co-morbidity survey. *American Journal of Orthopsychiatry, 66* (1), 17–31.

Kieckhefer, G. M., & Dinno, N. (1992, Fall). Neurodevelopmental outcomes and family needs of infants born mothers with a history of substance abuse. *Newsletter of the Clearinghouse for Drug Exposed Children, 3* (4), 1, 3, 5.

Knight, D., & Wadsworth, D. (1993). Physically challenged students: Inclusion classrooms. *Journal of the Association for Childhood Education International, 69* (4), 211–215.

Kolb, B., & Whishaw, I. Q. (1985). *Fundamentals of human neuropsychology* (2nd ed.). New York, NY: W. H. Freeman.

Kopera-Frye, K., Dehaene, S., & Streissguth, A. P. (1996). Impairments of number processing induced by prenatal alcohol exposure. *Neuropsychologia, 34* (12), 1187–1196.

Koren, G., Nulman, I., Chudley, A. E., & Loocke, C. (2003). Fetal alcohol spectrum disorder. *Canadian Medical Association Journal, 169* (11), 1181–1186.

Korkman, M., Kettunen, S., & Autti-Ramo, I. (2003). Neurocognitive impairment in early adolescence following prenatal alcohol exposure of varying duration. *Child Neuropsychology, 9* (2), 117–118.

Kosofsky, B. E., & Wilkins, A. S. (1998). A mouse model of transplacental cocaine exposure: Clinical implications for exposed infants and children. *Annals of the New York Academy of Sciences, 846,* 248–261.

Kudo, T. (1984). The effect of semantic plausibility on sentence comprehension in aphasia. *Brain and Language, 21* (2), 208–218.

Kuhn, C., Bero, L., Ignar, D., Lurie, S., & Field, E. (1987). Endocrine consequences of perinatal methadone exposure. In Friedman, D. P. & Clouet, D. H. (Eds.). *The role of neuroplasticity in the response to drugs.* NIDA Research Monograph 78, Rockville, MD: National Institute on Drug Abuse.

Lange, R. A., Cigarroa, R. G., Yancy, C. W., Willard, J. E., Popma, J. J., Sills, M. N., McBride, W., Kim, A. S., & Hills, L. D. (1989). Cocaine-induced coronary-artery vasoconstriction. *The New England Journal of Medicine, 321* (23), 1557–1562.

LeDoux, J. (2002). *Synaptic self: How our brains become who we are.* New York, Penguin.

Lemoine, P. (2003). The history of alcoholic fetopathies (1997). *J FAS Int, 1:e2, The Hospital for Sick Children.*

Lester, B. M., LaGasse, L., Seifer, R., Tronick, E. Z., Bauer, C. R., Shankaran, S., Bada, H., Wright, L. L., Smeriglio, V. L., Liu, J., Finnegan, L. P., & Maza, P. L. (2003). The maternal lifestyle study (MLS): Effects of prenatal cocaine and/or opiate exposure on auditory brain response at one month. *The Journal of Pediatrics, 142* (3), 279–285.

Lewis, B. A., Singer, L. T., Short, E. J., Minnes, S., Arendt, R., Weishampel, P., Klein, N., & Meeyoung, O. M. (2004). Four-year language outcomes of children exposed to cocaine in utero. *Neurotoxicology and Teratology, 26* (5), 617–627.

Lindsley, R. (1984, Spring). Learning about literacy: The children and me. *OAEYC Bulletin:* p. 11.

Little, R. E., & Sing C. F. (1986). Association of father's drinking and infant's birth weight. *New England Journal of Medicine, 314* (25), 1644–1645.

Luria, A. R. (1970a, March). The functional organization of the brain. *Scientific American, 222* (3), 66–78.

Luria, A. R. (1970b). *Traumatic aphasia: Its syndromes, psychology and treatment.* The Hague: Mouton.

MacGregor, S. N., Do, Keith, L. G., Bachicha, J. A., & Chasnoff, I. J. (1989). Cocaine abuse during pregnancy: Correlation between prenatal care and perinatal outcome. *Obstetrics and Gynecology, 74* (6), 882–885.

Magid, K., & McKelvey, C. A. (1987). *High risk: Children without a conscience.* New York, NY: Bantam Books.

Maguire, J. (1990). *Care and feeding of the brain: A guide to your gray matter.* New York, NY: Doubleday.

Mann, P. H., Suiter, P. A., & McClung, R. M. (1992). *A guide for educating mainstreamed students.* Boston, MA: Allyn and Bacon.

Maranto, G. (1984, May). The mind within the brain. *Discover,* pp. 34–35, 37, 40–43.

Martinez, M., & Roser, N. (1985). Read it again: The value of repeated readings during storytime. *Reading Teacher, 38* (8), 782–786.

Mattson, S. M., Riley, E. P., Gramling, L., Delis, D. C., & Jones, K. L. (1998). Neuropsychological comparison of alcohol-exposed children with or without physical features of fetal alcohol syndrome. *Neuropsychology, 12* (1), 146–153.

Mattson, S. N., & Riley, E. P. (2000). Parent ratings of behavior in children with heavy prenatal alcohol exposure and IQ-matched controls. *Alcoholism Clinical and Experimental Research, 24* (2), 226–231.

Mattson, S. N., & Riley, E. P. (1998). A review of the neurobehavioral deficits in children with fetal alcohol syndrome or prenatal exposure to alcohol. *Alcoholism: Clinical and Experimental Research, 22* (2), 279–294.

Mattson, S. N., & Roebuch, T. M. (2002). Acquisition and retention of verbal and nonverbal information in children with heavy prenatal alcohol exposure. *Alcoholism Clinical and Experimental Research, 26* (6), 875–882.

Mattson, S. N., Schoenfeld, A. M., & Riley, E. P. (2001). Teratogenic effects of alcohol on brain and behavior. *Alcohol Health and Research World, 25* (3), 185–191.

Mayes, L. (2003). Genetics of childhood disorders: LV. prenatal drug exposure. *Journal of the American Academy of Child and Adolescent Psychiatry, 42* (10), 1258–1261.

Mayes, L. C., Domenic, C., Suddhasatta, A., & Heping, Z. (2003). Developmental trajectories of cocaine-and-other-drug-exposed and non-cocaine-exposed children. *Journal of Developmental and Behavioral Pediatrics, 24* (5), 323–335.

Mayes, L. C., Granger, R. H., Bornstein, M. H., & Zuckerman, B. (1992). The problem of prenatal cocaine exposure: A rush to judgment. *Journal of the American Medical Association, 267* (3), 406–408.

McDaniel, M. A., & Kearney E. M. (1984). Optimal learning strategies and their spontaneous use: The importance of task-appropriate processing. *Memory and Cognition, 12* (4), 361–373.

McIntyre, C. K., Marriott, L. K., & Gold, P. E. (2003). Cooperation between memory systems: Acetylcholine release in the amygdala correlates positively with performance on a hippocampus-dependent task [articles]. *Behavioral Neuroscience, 117* (2), 320–326.

Mirochnick, M., Meyer, J., Frank, D. A., Cabral, H., Tronick, E. Z., & Zuckerman, B. (1997). Elevated plasma norepinephrine after in utero exposure to cocaine and marijuana. *Pediatrics, 99* (4), 555–559.

Mishkin, M., & Appenzeller, T. (1987, June). The anatomy of memory. *Scientific American, 256* (6), 80–89.

Monnot, M., Lovallo, W. R., Nixon, S. J., & Ross, E. (2002). Neurological basis of deficits in affective prosody comprehension among alcoholics and fetal alcohol-exposed adults. *The Journal of Neuropsychiatry and Clinical Neurosciences, 14,* 321–328.

Montori, V. M., Jaeschke, R., Schunemann, H. J., Bhandari, M., Brozek, J. L., Devereaux, P. J., & Guyatt, G. H. (2004). Users' guide to detecting misleading claims in clinical research reports. *British Medical Journal, 329* (7474), 1093–1096.

Moore, K. L., & Persaud, T. V. N. (1993). *The developing human: Clinically oriented embryology* (5th ed.). Philadelphia, PA: W. B. Saunders.

Morris, J S., deBonis, M., & Dolan, R. J. (2002). Human amygdala responses to fearful eyes. *NeuroImage, 17* (1), 214–222.

Morrow, C., Bandstra, E. S., Anthony, J. C., Ofir, A. Y, Xue, L., & Eyes, M. B. (2003). Influence of prenatal cocaine exposure on early language development: Longitudinal findings from four months to three years of age. *Journal of Developmental and Behavioral Pediatrics, 24* (1), 39–50.

Moskowitz, B. A. (1978, November). The acquisition of language. *Scientific American, 239* (5), 92–108.

Musto, D. F. (1991). Opium, cocaine and marijuana in American history. *Scientific American, 265* (1), 40–47.

Nader, K. (2003). Memory traces unbound. *Trends in Neurosciences, 26* (2), 65–72.

Nanson J. L., & Hiscock M.(1990). Attention deficits in children exposed to alcohol prenatally. *Alcoholism: Clinical and Experimental Research, 14* (5), 656–661.

Nelson, S., Lerner, E., Needlman, R., Salvator, A., & Singer, L. (2004). Cocaine, anemia, and neurodevelopmental outcomes in children: A longitudinal study. *Journal of Developmental and Behavioral Pediatrics, 25* (1), 1–9.

Nordstrom-Klee, B., Delaney-Black, V., Covington, C., Ager, J., & Sokol, R. (2002). Growth from birth onwards of children prenatally exposed to drugs: A literature review. *Neurotoxicology and Teratology, 24* (4), 481–488.

Norman, D. A. (1982). *Learning and memory.* San Francisco, CA: W. H. Freeman.

Norris, J. (1991). Providing developmentally appropriate intervention to infants and young children with handicaps. *Topics in Early Childhood Special Education, 11* (1), 21–35.

O'Connor, M. J., Kogan, N., & Findlay, R. (2002). Prenatal alcohol exposure and attachment behavior in children. *Alcoholism Clinical and Experimental Research, 26* (10), 1592–1602.

O'Connor, M. J., Shah, B, Whaley, S., Cronin, P., Gunderson, B., & Graham, J. (2002). Psychiatric illness in a clinical sample of children with prenatal alcohol exposure. *American Journal Drug Alcohol Abuse, 28* (4), 743–54.

O'Malley, K. D., (2003). Youth with comorbid disorders. In: Pumariega, A. J. & Winters, N. C. (eds.). *The Handbook of Child and Adolescent Systems of Care.* San Francisco: Jossy-Bass.

O'Shea, T. M., Klinepeter, K. L., Goldstein, D. J., Jackson, B. W., & Dillard, R. G. (1997). Survival and developmental disability in infants with birth weights of 501 to 800 grams, born between 1979 and 1994. *Pediatrics, 100* (6), 982–986.

Olson, H. C. (2002). Helping children with fetal alcohol syndrome and related conditions: A clinician's overview. In R. J. McMahon & R. D. Peters (Ed.). *The Effects of Parental Dysfunction on Children* (147–177). New York: Kluwer Academic/ Plenum.

Passaro, K. T., Little, R. E., Savitz, D. A., & Noss, J. (1998). Effect of paternal alcohol consumption before conception on infant birth weight. ALSPAC study team. Avon Longitudinal Study of Pregnancy and Childhood. *Teratology, 57* (6), 294–301.

Peters, H., & Theorell, C. J. (1991). Fetal and neonatal effects of maternal cocaine use. *Journal of Obstetric, Gynecologic, and Neonatal Nursing 20* (2), 121–126.

Pinker, S. (2000). *The language instinct.* New York: Perennial Classics.

Poitra, B. A., Marion, S., Dionne, M., Wilkie, E., Dauphinais, P., Wilkie-Pepion, M., Martsolf, J. T., Klug, M. G., & Burd, L. (2003). A school-based screening program for fetal alcohol syndrome. *Neurotoxicology and Teratology, 25* (6), 725–729.

Praisner, C. L. (2003). Attitudes of elementary school principals toward the inclusion of students with disabilities. *Council for Exceptional Children, 69* (12), 135–(11).

Pulsifer, M. B., Radonovich, K., Belcher, H. M. E., & Butz, A. M. (2004). Intelligence and school readiness in preschool children with prenatal drug exposure. *Child Neuropsychology, 10* (2), 89–101.

Quevedo, J., Sant'Anna, M. K., Madruga, M., Lovato, I., de-Paris, F., Kapczinski, F., Izquierdo, I., & Cahill, L. (2003). Differential effects of emotional arousal in short- and long-term memory in healthy adults. *Neurobiology of Learning and Memory, 79* (2), 132–135.

Rapin, I. (1988). Disorders of higher cerebral function in preschool children. *American Journal of Diseases of Children, 142* (10), 1119–1124.

Restak, R. (2003). *The new brain: How the modern age is rewiring your mind.* USA: Rodale.

Restak, R. M. (1979). *The brain: The last frontier.* New York, NY: Warner Books: 418.

Restak, R. M. (1988). *The mind.* New York, NY: Bantam Books: 123.

Reynolds, C. R. (1981). The neuropsychological basis of intelligence. In G. W. Hynd & J. E. Obrzut (Eds.). *Neuropsychological assessment and the school-age child* (pp. 87–124). New York, NY: Grune & Stratton.

Riley, E. P., Guerri, C., Calhoun, F., Charness, M. E., Foroud, T. M., Li, T. K., Mattson, S. N., May, P. A., & Warren, K. R. (2003). Prenatal alcohol exposure: Advancing knowledge through international collaborations. *Alcoholism Clinical and Experimental Research, 27* (1), 118–35.

Riley, E. P., Mattson, S. N., Li, T. K., Jacobson, S. W., Coles, C. D., Kodituwakku, P. W., Adnams, C. M., & Korkman, M. I. (2003). Neurobehavioral consequences of prenatal alcohol exposure: An international perspective. *Alcoholism Clinical and Experimental Research, 27* (2), 362–373.

Rimland, B. (1990). The non-urban alternative. *Autism Research Review International, 4* (3).

Rock, I. (1958, August). Repetition and learning. *Scientific American, 199* (2), 68–82.

Rodning, C., Beckwith, L., & Howard, J. (1989). Prenatal exposure to drugs and its influence on attachment. *Annals New York Academy of Sciences, 562,* 352–354

Roe, D. A., Little, B. B., Bawdon, R. E., & Gilstrap, L. C. (1990). Metabolism of cocaine by human placentas: Implications for fetal exposure. *American Journal of Obstetrics and Gynecology 163* (3), 715–718.

Roebuck, T. M., Mattson, S. N., & Riley, E. P. (2002). Interhemispheric transfer in children with heavy prenatal alcohol exposure. *Alcoholism Clinical and Experimental Research, 26* (12), 1863–1871.

Roit, M. L., & McKenzie, R. G. (1985). Disorders of written communication: An instructional priority for LD students. *Journal of Learning Disabilities, 18* (5), 258–260.

Rosenzweig, M. R., Bennett, E. L., & Diamond, M. C. (1972, February). Brain changes in response to experience. *Scientific American, 226* (2), 22–29.

Sachs, B., & Hall, L. A. (1991, Dec. 8). Maladaptive mother-child relationships: A pilot study. *Public Health Nursing, 4,* 226–233.

Savitz, D. A., Zhang, J., Schwingl, P., & John, E. M. (1992). Association of paternal alcohol use with gestational age and birth weight. *Teratology, 46,* 465–471.

Schacter, D. L. (2001). *The seven sins of memory: How the mind forgets and remembers.* New York, Houghton Mifflin.

Schacter, D. L. (1982). *Stranger behind the engram: Theories of memory and the psychology of science.* Hillsdale, NJ: Lawrence Erlbaum Associates.

Schneider, J. W., & Chasnoff, I. J. (1987). Cocaine abuse during pregnancy: Its effects on infant motor development—A clinical perspective. *Topics in Acute Care and Trauma Rehabilitation, 2* (1), 59–69.

Schneider, J. W., & Chasnoff, I. J. (1992). Motor assessment of cocaine/polydrug exposed infants at age 4 months. *Neurotoxicology and Teratology, 14* (2), 97–101.

Schneider, J. W., Lee, W., & Chasnoff, I. J. (1988). Field testing of the movement assessment of infants. *Physical Therapy, 68* (3), 321–327.

Schonfeld, A. M., Mattson, S. N., Lang, A. R., Delis, D. C., & Riley, E. P. (2001). Verbal and nonverbal fluency in children with heavy prenatal alcohol exposure. *Journal of Studies on Alcohol, 62* (2), 239–246.

Schroder, M. D., Snyder, P. J., Sielski, I., & Mayes, L. (2004). Impaired performance of children exposed in utero to cocaine on a novel test of visuospatial working memory. *Brain and Cognition, 55* (2), 409–412.

Schuler, M. E., Nair, P., & Kettinger, L. (2003). Drug-exposed infants and developmental outcome: Effects of a home intervention and ongoing maternal drug use. *Archives of Pediatric Adolescent Medicine, 157* (2), 133–138.

Shatz, C. J. (1992, September). The developing brain. *Scientific American, 267* (3), 60–67.

Shaywitz, S. E., & Shaywitz, B. A. (2003). Dyslexia (specific reading disability). *Pediatrics in Review, 24,* 147–153.

Singer, L. T., Minnes, S., Short, E., Arendt, R., Farkas, K., Lewis, B., Klein, N., Russ, S., Min, M. O., & Kirchner, H. L. (2004). Cognitive outcomes of preschool children with prenatal cocaine exposure. *The Journal of the American Medical Association, 291* (20), 2448–2456.

Singer, L. T., Salvator, A., Arendt, R., Minnes, S., Farkas, K., & Kliegman, R. (2002). Effects of cocaine/polydrug exposure and maternal psychological distress on infant birth outcomes. *Neurotoxicology and Teratology, 24* (2), 127–135.

Singer, L. T., Arendt, R., Minnes, S., Farkas, K., Salvator, A., Kirchner, H., Lester, H., & Kliegman, R. (2002). Cognitive and motor outcomes of cocaine-exposed infants. *Journal of the American Medical Association, 287* (15), 1952–1960.

Singer, L. T., Arendt, R., Minnes, S., Salvator, A., Siegel, A. C., & Lewis, B. A. (2001). Developing language skills of cocaine-exposed infants. *Pediatrics, 107* (5), 1057–1064.

Singer, L., Farkas, K., & Kliegman, R. (1992). Childhood medical and behavioral consequences of maternal cocaine use. *Journal of Pediatric Psychology, 17* (4), 389–406.

Singer, L. T., Garber, R., & Kliegman, R. (1991). Neurobehavioral sequelae of fetal cocaine exposure. *The Journal of Pediatrics, 119* (4), 667–672.

Somerville, J. (1989 June 16). Cocaine babies: Issue for the courts? *American Medical News:* pp. 9, 41–42.

Sowell, E. R., Thompson, P. M., Mattson, S. N., Tessner, K. D., Jernigan, T. L., Riley, E. P., & Toga, A. W. (2002). Regional brain shape abnormalities persist into adolescence after heavy prenatal alcohol exposure. *Cerebral Cortex, 12* (8), 856–865.

Sowell, E. R., Thompson, P. M., Peterson, B. S., Mattson, S. N., Welcome, S. E., Henkenius, A. L., Riley, E. P., Jernigan, T. L., & Toga, A. W. (2002). Mapping cortical gray matter asymmetry patterns in adolescents with heavy prenatal alcohol exposure. *NeuroImage, 17,* 1807–1819.

Sowell, E. R., Mattson, S. N., Thompson, P. M., Jernigan, T. L., Riley, E. P., & Toga, A. W. (2001). Mapping callosal morphology and cognitive correlates: Effects of heavy prenatal alcohol exposure. *Neurology, 57* (2), 235–244.

Spaide, R. F. (1990). Shaken baby syndrome. *American Family Physician, 41* (4), 1145–1152.

Spear, L. P., Silveri, M. M., Casale, M., Katovic, N. M., Campbell, J. O., & Douglas, L. A. (2002). Cocaine and development: A retrospective perspective. *Neurotoxicology and Teratology, 24* (3), 321–327.

Spear, N. E. (1984). Ecologically determined dispositions control the ontogeny of learning and memory. In R. Kail & E. Spear (Eds.), *Comparative perspectives on the development of memory* (pp. 325–358). Hillsdales, NJ: Lawrence Erlbaum Associates.

Squire, L. R., & Kandel, E. R. (1999). *Memory: From mind to molecules.* New York: Henry Holt.

Squire, L. R. (1986). Mechanisms of memory. *Science, 232* (4758), 1612–1619.

Stanley, S. (1992). *Maternity ward: Behind the scenes at a big city hospital.* New York, NY: William Morrow: 145.

Steinhausen, H., Willms, J., Metzke, C. W., & Spohr, H. (2003). Behavioural phenotype in foetal alcohol syndrome and foetal alcohol effects. *Developmental Medicine and Child Neurology, 45* (3), 179–182.

Steinmetz, G. (1992, Feb.). The preventable tragedy: Fetal alcohol syndrome. *National Geographic, 181* (2), 36–39.

Stoler, J. M, & Holmes, L. B. (2000) Under-recognition of prenatal alcohol effects in infants of known alcohol abusing women. *Obstetrical and Gynecological Survey, 55* (5), 278–279.

Streissguth, A. P., Bookstein, F. L., Barr, H. M., Sampson, P. D., O'Malley, K., & Young, J. K. (2004). Risk factors for adverse life outcomes in fetal alcohol syndrome and fetal alcohol effects. *Journal of Developmental and Behavioral Pediatrics, 25* (4), 228–238.

Streissguth, A. P., & O'Malley, K. (2000). Neuropsychiatric implications and long-term consequences of fetal alcohol spectrum disorders. *Seminars in Clinical Neuropsychiatry, 5* (3), 177–190.

Streissguth, A. P., & Kanter, K. (Eds). (1999). *The challenge of fetal alcohol syndrome: Overcoming secondary disabilities.* Seattle: University of Washington Press.

Streissguth, A. P., Randels, S. P., & Smith, D. F. (1991b). A test-retest study of intelligence in patients with fetal alcohol syndrome: Implications for care. *Journal of the American Academy of Child and Adolescence Psychiatry, 30* (4), 584–587.

Streissguth, A. P., Aase, J. M., Clarren, S. K., Randels, S. P., LaDue, R. A., & Smith, D. F. (1991a). Fetal alcohol syndrome in adolescents and adults. *The Journal of the American Medical Association, 265* (15), 1961–1967.

Streissguth, A. P., Sampson, P. D., & Barr, H. M. (1989). Neurobehavioral dose-response effects of prenatal alcohol exposure in humans from infancy to adulthood. *Annals New York Academy of Sciences, 562,* 145–158.

Streissguth, A. P., LaDue, R. A., & Randels, S. P. (1988). *A manual on adolescents and adults with fetal alcohol syndrome with special reference to American Indians.* (Contract No. 240-83-0035 and 243-88-0166). Washington, DC: U.S. Department of Health and Human Services.

Streissguth, A. P. (1987, Sept.). FAS only the tip of the iceberg. *U.S. Journal of Drug and Alcohol Dependence:* p.8.

Stromland, K., & Hellstrom, M. (1996). Fetal alcohol syndrome—An ophthalmological and socioeducational prospective study. *Pediatrics, 97* (6), 845–850.

Swayze, V. W., Johnson, V. P., Hanson, J. W., Piven, J., Sato, Y., Giedd, J. N., Mosnik, D., & Andreasen, N. C. (1997). Magnetic resonance imaging of brain anomalies in fetal alcohol syndrome. *Pediatrics, 99* (2), 232–240.

Sylwester, R. (1986, Summer). Learning about learning: The neurosciences and the education profession. *Educational Horizons:* 162–167.

Tabor, B. L., Soffici, A. R., Smith-Wallace, T., Yonekura, M. L. (1991). The effect of maternal cocaine use on the fetus: Changes in antepartum fetal heart rate tracings. *American Journal of Obstetrics and Gynecology, 165* (5), 1278–1281.

Tedder, J. L. (1991). Using the Brazelton Neonatal Assessment Scale to facilitate the parent-infant relationship in a primary care setting. *Nurse Practitioner, 16* (3), 26–30, 35–36.

Thompson, R. F. (1986). The neurobiology of learning and memory. *Science, 233* (4767), 941–947.

Tronick, E. Z., Frank, D. A., Cabral, H., Mirochnick, M., & Zuckerman, B. (1996). Late dose-response effects of prenatal cocaine exposure on newborn neurobehavioral performance. *Pediatrics, 98* (1), 76–83.

Trost, C. (1989, Dec. 27). As drug babies grow older, schools strive to meet their needs. *The Wall Street Journal:* pp. Sec.A 1–2.

Van de Bor, M., Walther, F. J. & Ebrahimi, M. (1990). Decreased cardiac output in infants of mothers who abused cocaine. *Pediatrics, 85* (1), 30–32.

Viljoen, D. L., Carr, L. G., Foroud, T. M., Brooke, L., Ramsay, M., & Li, T. K. (2001). Alcohol Dehydrogenase-2*2 Allele is associated with decreased prevalence of fetal alcohol syndrome in the mixed-ancestry population of the Western Cape Province, South Africa. *Alcoholism Clinical and Experimental Research, 25* (12), 1719–1722.

Viscarello, R. R., Ferguson, D. D., Nores, J., & Hobbins, J. C. (1992). Limb-body wall complex associated with cocaine abuse: Further evidence of cocaine's teratogenicity. *Obstetrics and Gynecology, 80* (3), 523–526.

Volpe, J. J. (1992). Effect of cocaine use on the fetus. *The New England Journal of Medicine, 327* (6), 399–405.

Wass, T. S., Simmons, R. W., Thomas, J. D., & Riley, E. P. (2002). Timing accuracy and variability in children with prenatal exposure to alcohol. *Alcoholism Clinical and Experimental Research, 26* (12), 1887–1896.

Weidner, W. E., & Jinks, A. F. G. (1983). The effects of single versus combined cue presentations on picture naming by aphasic adults. *Journal of Communication Disorders, 16,* 111–121.

Whaley, S. E., O'Connor, M. J., & Gunderson, B. (2001). Comparison of the adaptive functioning of children prenatally exposed to alcohol to a nonexposed clinical sample. *Alcoholism Clinical and Experimental Research, 25* (7), 1018–1024.

White, M., & Miller, S. R. (1983). Dyslexia: A term in search of a definition. *The Journal of Special Education, 17* (1), 5–10.

Whitman, T. L., Spence, B. H., & Maxwell, S. (1987). A comparison of external and self-instructional teaching formats with mentally retarded adults in a vocational training setting. *Research in Developmental Disabilities, 8* (3), 371–388.

Willford, J. A., Richardson, G. A., Leech, S. L., & Day, N. L. (2004). Verbal and visuospatial learning and memory function in children with moderate prenatal alcohol exposure. *Alcoholism Clinical and Experimental Research, 28* (3), 497–507.

Woods, J. R., Plessinger, M. A., & Clark, K. E. (1987). Effect of cocaine on uterine blood flow and fetal oxygenation. *Journal of the American Medical Association, 257* (7), 957–961.

Wright, B., & Garrett, M. (1984). Lexical decision in sentences: Effects of syntactic structure. *Memory and Cognition, 12* (1), 31–45.

INDEX

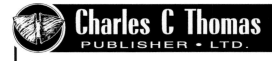

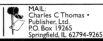